American Plastic

American Plastic

Boob Jobs,
Credit Cards,
and Our Quest for Perfection

Laurie Essig

BEACON PRESS BOSTON

Beacon Press
25 Beacon Street
Boston, Massachusetts 02108-2892
www.beacon.org

Beacon Press books
are published under the auspices of
the Unitarian Universalist Association of Congregations.

13 12 11 10   8 7 6 5 4 3 2 1

This book is printed on acid-free paper that meets the uncoated paper ANSI/NISO
specifications for permanence as revised in 1992.

Text design by Jody Hanson at Wilsted & Taylor Publishing Services

Library of Congress Cataloging-in-Publication Data
Essig, Laurie.
  American plastic : boob jobs, credit cards, and our quest for perfection / Laurie Essig.
    p. cm.
  Includes bibliographical references and index.
  ISBN 978-0-8070-0055-7 (hardcover : alk. paper) 1. Credit cards—United States.
2. Credit—United States. 3. Surgery, Plastic—Social aspects. 4. Surgery, Plastic—
Moral and ethical aspects. I. Title.
  HG3755.8.U6E87 2010
  332.7'650973—dc22   2010007765

*This book is dedicated to Willa and Georgia,
the two most beautiful people I know.*

Author's Note

To protect the innocent and the guilty and all the rest of us, the names and identifying features of individuals profiled or interviewed herein have been changed, except as noted. Some stories reflect composites of individuals and/or conversations. Sources who agreed to go on the record, as well as published sources, are clearly identified by name and affiliation or professional capacity.

Contents

Introduction

In October of 2008 I delivered a lecture at the British Museum. I had been invited to give the talk as part of a series on health and human society called "Making Things Better," sponsored by University College London. The British Museum is kind of a big deal, at least for me. After all, it was here that Karl Marx spent years of his life, sitting in the Reading Room, figuring out how capitalism worked. I myself spent months preparing for my talk. I came up with the perfect images, the perfect PowerPoint, the perfect title. The subject of the talk, the relationship between cosmetic surgery and pornography, was titillating and meant to attract a crowd. But as I walked up the imposing steps of the museum and the shadows of the enormous Greek Revival columns swept over me, I couldn't help but feel as if I didn't deserve to be there. Marx told us that the philosophers had merely interpreted the world; the point was to change it. I suddenly felt nervous, that my talk was not good enough, not important enough, for this illustrious place setting, with its 250 years of distinguished history and its more than 7 million objects. I began to panic.

London itself was in a panic. Every time I turned on the BBC, commentators with a hysterical edge to their voices blathered on about the "credit crunch" as if nuclear annihilation had arrived. Is this it? Is this the big one? Will we survive? Banks were failing; retirements were vanishing overnight. I stood at the lectern that evening and announced that the advertised talk would not take place. "I will not be discussing pornography and plastic surgery tonight," I said, my own voice verging on hysteria. Groans emanated from a few audience members who were hoping for prurient images. I felt even more nervous as I cleared my throat and announced, "Instead, I will explain the collapse of the American economy through cosmetic surgery." This time there were snickers. Perhaps even a guffaw. How absurd. How could something as trivial as boob jobs possibly explain the collapse of the American economy and the ensuing credit crunch in the UK? The answer is unexpectedly interesting: it's a story about greed, politics, and desire. Ultimately, it's a story about plastic.

Do you remember that scene from *The Graduate,* when Walter Brooke's character, Mr. McGuire, gives the young Ben Braddock, played by Dustin Hoffman, the following advice?

> I want to say one word to you. Just one word . . . Are you listening? . . . *Plastics.*

I think that Mr. McGuire was right. "Plastics" is the one word we need to listen to. The more I listen to plastic, the more I realize how crucial it is. I would argue that one cannot understand America, and therefore the world today, without understanding plastic.

The story of plastic is not an easy one to tell. Rather than existing in linear time, it melts back and forth between past and present, with a few glimpses of what the future will bring. I began paying attention to the story of plastic about a decade ago. A friend and I were running through Brooklyn's Prospect Park. Allie, who had just broken up with her longtime partner, announced: "I'm thinking of getting my boobs done."

I stopped dead in my tracks. "What?" I panted. "What are you going to do to them?"

"They're so small," she explained. "I think if they were bigger I wouldn't be so scared of being alone."

This statement shocked me at the time. How would bigger breasts make Allie more secure? How would spending thousands of dollars on her surface change what she was feeling inside? How could my educated, professional, feminist, and yes, lesbian friend believe that bigger boobs would improve her sense of well-being?

Last year, I was having an equally illogical conversation with another friend, Sam, but this time it was financial, not romantic, insecurity that drove her to plastic. I was sitting in the cozy kitchen of her home in a rural New England town, a sort of modern cabin, set in the woods near a stream. Sam is a beautiful woman, approaching forty. Her daughter, Lee, who is blond and big-eyed and smart like her mom, was hanging onto her mother's slim waist. Sam had just finished college. As the mother of two young children, she had won a scholarship to a prestigious school, and had somehow managed to run her household, help with her husband's business, and be an honor roll co-ed. Sam is the first one in her family to get a college degree. We talked about how she had finally achieved her goals, and I assumed she was feeling something like satisfaction.

But like Allie, Sam was unhappy. It was not her marriage or even the fact that her son was torturing bullfrogs outside their quaint home that gnawed away at the perfection of her life. It was the size of her boobs. "They're too small," she lamented. All her life, she'd wanted bigger breasts, and now that she had achieved so much, she deserved to get what she really wanted. Unfortunately, getting bigger boobs was a difficult decision for Sam, since, like most Americans, her family had no savings and spent more than their net income every year, meaning they had not just "good" debt, like a mortgage, but the bad, plastic-money kind. Since breast implants cost about $8,000, she could not easily afford them. None of these facts shaped the logic with which Sam operated. She went into the plastic surgeon's office to talk about payment plans and other options. But what, exactly, would drive this very driven woman to plastic surgery? Even after nearly two decades together, her husband and she had a strong sexual and emotional connection. Yet Sam's romantic security did not necessarily translate into economic security. Sam was stressed, overworked, and quite honestly scared about her financial future. There was nothing to do but get bigger boobs.

Sam and Allie are part of a growing number of Americans who are turning to cosmetic surgery as a path to happiness. It is easy to judge them, but only if we ignore the reality of our own lives. Nearly all of us are engaged in the project of "first impressions." We diet and exercise and dye our hair and buy new clothes and wax our eyebrows and any other offending body hair we might have. We focus not just on the plastic shell of our bodies, but on the shells of our homes and cars and technologies. Even if you don't crave a perfect body, you fantasize about the perfect kitchen, or sports car, or garden. And even if you have avoided spending a good chunk of your time and money on such aesthetic pursuits, perhaps you're obsessed by trying to produce the perfectly groomed and trained child. In other words, for most Americans, the difference between those of us who get cosmetic surgery and those who don't is one of focus, not of degree or kind.

Besides, Sam and Allie are deeper than most of us. Sam's a spiritual woman who recently returned from a trip volunteering in an orphanage in a desperately poor country. Allie is committed to educating her children in a progressive Jewish tradition. And Sam and Allie are healthier than most of us; they don't drink or smoke, they exercise regularly and eat sensibly. But their breasts, well, they're "ordinary" and possibly even "small." They just don't feel as beautiful as they want to feel, and the surgeons promise to make them feel better. We all want to feel better. So many of us inhabit bodies that we don't love. So many of us just want to know how to fix ourselves. So many of us perceive the problems outside of us—the wars, the economy, the environment—as beyond our control or influence. We wish the world were different. We wish we were different. The solution, it seems, is plastic.

In the first decade of the twenty-first century, despite terrorist attacks, wars without end, and economic collapse, Americans
had more than 10 million surgical and nonsurgical cosmetic
procedures every year. Surgical procedures include things like
liposuction and facelifts; nonsurgical procedures include Botox
injections and laser resurfacing of the skin. According to the
American Society for Aesthetic Plastic Surgery, in the past ten
years, there has been a 465 percent increase in the total number
of cosmetic procedures. Americans spend just under $12.5 bil-
lion on cosmetic procedures annually.[1] That's more than twice
what is spent each year in the world on basic education. It is, in
other words, a lot of money.

It is now no longer a question of why someone would go under
the knife, but rather, why not? Plastic surgery is increasingly seen
as an acceptable and even desirable undertaking. A 2008 survey
shows Americans feeling more positive about plastic surgery than
they did just ten years ago. This change from seeing plastic surgery as a luxury to seeing it as "the answer" to almost everything,
from aging to divorce to loss of libido, didn't happen by itself.
Our desire for plastic is the result of massive shifts in our culture
and our economy that affect us all. Plastic money covered up the
fact that most of us were getting poorer while a few of us were getting richer. Plastic surgery was paid for by that plastic money, but
so were a lot of other things. We became obsessed with creating
perfectly smooth and shiny plastic surfaces.

Nearly all Americans have been trapped by the promise of
plastic. It doesn't matter whether you have ever considered cosmetic surgery yourself or even known anyone who has, chances
are you've assumed debt in order to create a more perfect future.
There's something alluring about it. Perfection is coming, just
down the road, if only you'll buy this "new and improved" version now. "Perfect" seems to have first appeared as an advertising
catchword in the 1920s, as a way to get people to ignore the cost
of an item. And perfection is priceless—immediate on the one

hand but a promise deferred on the other. Simply put, one cannot get enough.[2] The promise of perfection reappeared with the opening up of plastic money in the 1980s. As wealth became concentrated in the top 20 percent of Americans, the rest of us took on debt to get the perfect future we were promised. The result was a perfect storm of greed and desire.

The Perfect Storm

In 1978 the world changed and, indeed, my world changed with it. That the world and I changed together is no accident; it was plastic that transformed us, plastic money and plastic selves. I was thirteen in 1978. Looking back from my forties, I am struck by how historical, economic, legal, and personal forces came together in such a seemingly predetermined way, as if we had no choice but to become plastic. Perhaps there really is a higher power, one made of plastic and with a seriously perverse sense of humor, running things. It certainly seems that way now.

In April of 1978, the TV show *Dallas* made its debut. For the first time, Americans could watch, desire, and imitate the lifestyles of the rich and famous Ewings, as opposed to the far more middle- and even working-class Cleavers and Bunkers who had populated prime time in the first decades of television. And watch the Ewings we did. Sitting next to my mother on a shabby couch in a shabby home snuggled between a pizzeria parking lot and the railroad tracks, we were captivated by the intrigues of these fictional Texas oil families. More than the twists and turns of the melodramatic plot, we tuned in to see their things: their unbelievably nice homes and cars and clothes. Money—big money—came to appear as normal and attainable as the Texas ladies' big hair and their men's big hats.

A few months after *Dallas* debuted, I went school shopping with my father. My father was middle class, and like most middle-class Americans at the time, he had a credit card given to him by his bank that had a very low interest rate and a limit that corresponded to his bank account. The child of divorce, I was growing up anything but middle class. In fact, I'd never seen a credit card up until that point. It seemed like magic to me that I could buy things without paying for them. I usually purchased my clothes at discount stores like Woolworth's, often putting them on layaway, paying them off with $5 a month cash, hard-earned from babysitting and bussing tables at the pizzeria next door. My father took me to the far more upscale Bloomingdale's, handed me the card, and told me to have fun. "Fun" is not the word for the ecstasy I felt as I touched, perhaps for the first time, the rich materials of the upper classes. I still remember the plush feel of a velour pullover and thick tweed jacket I purchased with the magic plastic money. How different it was from the shiny, plastic-feeling clothes they sold at Woolworth's. Running around department stores, charging clothes that would transform me from "poor" to "rich" in the eyes of my classmates and the world, I had my first taste of the power of MasterCard.

In December of the same year, the United States Supreme Court handed down the Marquette Bank decision, which effectively ended anti-usury laws by allowing banks to export their credit card operations to states without such laws. This meant that banks could start charging higher and higher interest rates and thus take on riskier and riskier customers for their credit cards. It also meant that other Americans like me, Americans who could ill afford the lush fabrics and natty tweeds I charged to my father's account, could also transform their wardrobes, and possibly their lives.

After 1978, plastic enabled Americans to live more and more lavish lifestyles—at whatever interest rate the market could bear. As if this magical coincidence wasn't enough, the next year, Ronald Reagan was elected president and "Reaganomics," which gave money to the rich in hopes it would "trickle down" to the poor, became official economic policy. As a result, Americans went further into debt as they made less money but spent more. Nearly three decades later, most Americans are worse off. Yet because of our cultural beliefs about wealth, like "pulling yourself up by your bootstraps," we have looked to individual solutions to economic insecurity rather than structural ones. Buying boobs, clothes, cars, even an education with plastic is now the well-worn path to the American dream of a better life.

According to Juliet Schor, author of *The Overspent American,* "Throughout the 1980s and 1990s, most middle class Americans were acquiring at a greater rate than any previous generation of the middle class. And their buying was more upscale."[3] Plastic surgery has become another "must have," akin to designer clothes and Caribbean vacations. This ever-expanding sense of need and desire is one of the major reasons the average American household debt stands at about 124 percent of after-tax income. It's why Americans pay $50 billion in finance charges per year and carry an average of $8,562 in credit card debt. Over a million credit card holders declared bankruptcy in 2008.[4] Schor notes that Americans spend 70 percent more now than they did in 1979, when in fact most Americans make less.

But many of us want more than a new wardrobe or an expensive meal. We want more than the luxurious lifestyle of the Ewings and the Reagans. We want to *look* like the rich as well as live like them. How lucky for our oversized desires and declining income that it was also at the exact moment we began to desire the *Lifestyles of the Rich and Famous* that plastic money and plastic surgery became increasingly available to the masses. A 2005 poll conducted by the American Society of Plastic Surgeons found that 30 percent of plastic surgery patients earned less than $30,000 a year while another 41 percent earned between $31,000 and $60,000.[5] Plastic surgery, once only for the wealthiest Americans, is now available to the rest of us. This makes sense when we put plastic surgery alongside a variety of economic and cultural trends occurring over the past two decades.

In other words, despite what some audience members at my

British Museum talk may have thought, it's not completely ridiculous to suggest that the credit crunch in the UK and the collapse of the economy in the United States can be explained through boob jobs. It may seem like something of a schizophrenic map, linking plastic beauty to plastic money to a political ideology of unregulated greed and a culture of worshiping the rich. But I know there are connections, the routes are well traveled, and the map is not just in my head, but written on the bodies and in the bank accounts of average Americans. I first realized that it was all connected by accident.

In 2004 I began to interview a group of young transgender men about their lives. Most of the young men had undergone breast-reassignment surgery, a cosmetic procedure where fatty tissue is suctioned from the breasts to flatten them, and the nipple is repositioned higher on the chest to make it appear more "masculine." The procedure costs somewhere between $6,000 and $8,000. I was surprised at the ability of these young people to pay for such a procedure, since most of them were recent college graduates with low-paying jobs. "Oh, it's easy," one young man assured me. "You just go into a cosmetic surgeon's office and there are all these credit companies and you just sign on the dotted line. Even if you have huge credit card debt and student loans, like me, they'll loan you the money."

As soon as I got home, I did a Web search on "cosmetic surgery" and "credit." Literally hundreds of sites came up, offering me money to make myself beautiful. As I dug deeper, I discovered that the vast majority of cosmetic surgery is paid for on credit. Most people getting cosmetic surgery are not rich, and a good number of them are poor. They're getting plastic surgery with plastic money at interest rates as high as 28 percent. In other words, people are taking on huge amounts of debt to reshape their bodies. This debt is not significantly different from the subprime mortgages people took on in the hopes of finally entering the middle class through the tried-and-true path of homeownership. It is the plastic promise of a better future through plastic money. It is a promise, as we now understand, that did not lead to a better life for most of us, unless we were the ones collecting interest payments on other peoples' dreams.

Fast-forward a few years. On a hot, late spring afternoon in 2007 I did something I had never done before and will probably never do again. I locked myself into my stuffy office in an old stone building on the picturesque college campus in Vermont where I teach. I rolled up my sleeves, kicked off my shoes, and waited for my phone to ring at the designated time. After initial introductions with the two men at the other end, two investment bankers from Wachovia, I began to advise them on the future of the American economy. I told them that the U.S. economy could not sustain its level of debt indefinitely and that it might be six months and it might be six years, but a serious downturn was inevitable. I uttered this incredibly sage advice just days before the official start of the "crash," as subprime mortgages led the way to the current recession. It is surprising that these bankers were asking me about the economy. It is even more surprising that I was right. I am a writer and a sociologist, not an economist. I don't really know anything about money. The truth is that I have never even tried to balance a checkbook, and I am more or less unable to do anything more mathematical than calculate a tip for my double latte. But I know a lot about plastic, and that's why the investment bankers called me, and that's why, by gazing into my plastic ball, I foresaw the future of the American economy and, I think, divined an important truth about American society.

Plastic Is Modern

American society, like plastic, is modern. As a variety of social critics have pointed out, what distinguishes modern societies from premodern ones is the internalization of power. In other words, back in the day, if the king wished to express the state's power, he chopped off a few heads. With modernity (and capitalism), power was no longer expressed through punishment of the body, but through its discipline. Not only are we moderns highly disciplined bodies, willing to go under the knife in order to show our loyalty to the order, but we inhabit bodies that represent our social status. As sociologist Pierre Bourdieu showed us, bodies are habituated in particular forms of power. A lifetime of habits (what Bourdieu calls *habitus*) produce our bodies as living illustrations of social power. Simply put, upper-class bodies look different from working-class ones; male bodies are inhabited differently than female ones. Social power is written on the physical body not because of innate genetics, but because of economic and cultural ideologies. Red meat is good/red meat is unhealthy; manual labor/daily yoga; cheap food/organic food; biggest breast implants possible/"natural-looking" breast implants. Taste is "a virtue made of necessity which continuously transforms necessity into virtue. . . . Through taste, an agent has what he likes because he likes what he has."[6]

Certain people have more of a "taste" for plastic surgery. Plastic surgery is not randomly distributed throughout the population. Plastic surgery is usually about the ordinary ugliness of women's bodies,[7] particularly middle-class, middle-aged, white women's bodies. Women had nearly 10.7 million cosmetic procedures in 2004, 90 percent of the total. Of these, 45 percent were between the ages of thirty-five and fifty and another 25 percent between fifty-one and sixty-four. That is, most of these women were middle-aged. Most were also white, about 80 percent[8] (versus 69 percent of the U.S. population). It is primarily the white and maternal body that seeks perfection in plastic surgery. Aging bodies, especially those of aging white women, elicit disgust. Think about what Rush Limbaugh famously asked in 2007, during Hillary Clinton's run for president: "Will Americans want to watch a woman get older before their eyes on a daily basis?" The answer for Rush and no doubt for a good number of Americans was No! A woman aging in front of our very eyes is just too revolting to witness.[9] Although the number of young people getting cosmetic surgery is increasing, the majority of people getting it are decidedly "aging."

Working-class bodies, which tend to be larger and have less access to things like braces for straight teeth or dermatologists for smooth skin, also elicit more disgust than the smooth, pampered bodies of the upper classes. That's why "gross" and "disgusting" bodies, often not fully clothed, are paraded around daytime TV, eliciting groans of "Ewww!" from the audience. Of course, about 20 percent of the people getting "work" done are of color, with 8 percent of the patients Hispanic, 6 percent African American, and 4 percent Asian American. Cosmetic surgery has always also been about making people "whiter," which is why its first customers in the United States were usually the "not quite white" Irish and Jews.

Certain bodies have more of a taste for plastic surgery than others, but at this point, most Americans have a taste for perfection. The mass internalization of the impossible project of perfection creates a feeling of disgust or even shock at the imperfect human body. Since we all exist in human bodies that are imperfect, we are all in a state of shock, either at our own bodies or the bodies of others. A population that is in shock, as Naomi Klein pointed out in *The Shock Doctrine,* is a population easily manipulated. For Klein, a population can be shocked into quiescence by a natural disaster or a murderous dictator who imprisons, tortures, and even murders anyone who might resist.[10] But what if the shock comes in a more personal, more internalized, more modern form? What if the shock we feel is at our own disgusting, shockingly imperfect bodies? And what if we are so shocked by our imperfect bodies that we are willing to give anything to find relief? What if modernity shocked us into plastic and now we're all paying the price, some of us paying in pounds of flesh as well as dollars and cents?

Are We There Yet? The Limits of Plastic

As I write this, the U.S. government is trying to save our plastic nation. In 2009 the American Recovery and Reinvestment Act pumped nearly $800 billion into the U.S. economy in hopes that the collective weight of bad debt would not take down the entire country, and with it the world. It remains to be seen whether or not the United States will recover from the weight of plastic money. According to the *American Heritage Dictionary,* "plastic" is that which is "capable of being shaped or formed . . . having the qualities of sculpture; well-formed . . . easily influenced . . . capable of undergoing continuous deformation without rupture or relaxation . . . marked by artificiality or superficiality . . . of or obtained by means of credit cards."

In case you haven't noticed, we Americans are increasingly becoming all these things: made of plastic, shaped by plastic, fake like plastic, deformed by plastic, made beautiful by plastic, paid for by plastic. We are living in a plastic time and place. How did we get here? The answers are both universal and particularly American. We got here because humans have always rewarded those seen as beautiful. We got here because technologies developed that allowed us to reshape the body. We got here because we live in a filmic age and looking good in two-dimensional space is not only desired, but also increasingly necessary.

We also got here because of our very American spirit. At the core of the American ethic is the idea that we are infinitely plastic; that we can always make our lives and ourselves better and maybe even the world a better place if we just work hard enough. Not enough wealth to go around? Go West! Feeling panicked about living in the nuclear age? Get therapy! Can't afford to buy a decent home? Get a no-money-down mortgage! Let's do it ourselves! Collapsing economy, crumbling bridges and roads, no health insurance, an environmental crisis the likes of which the world has never seen before? No problem, all we need to do is help ourselves become better, stronger, more able to cope, more, for lack of a better term, American. This can-do response to larger structural problems is at the heart of who we are as a people.

Unfortunately, a belief that we can keep improving ourselves forever and ever cannot actually counter the organized greed that has made most Americans poorer in the past thirty years and a select few of us much richer. There's been a wholesale shift in wealth in this country, in large part because the government stepped back from protecting ordinary Americans from extraordinary amounts of credit and debt. We are, as individuals and as a nation, debtors with an inability to pay the interest due, let alone put anything away for what is an increasingly insecure future.

Oddly enough, as concerned as some of us might be about plastic money and the trouble it's gotten us into, we continue to be obsessed about our boobs, our wrinkles, and the fat that has accumulated on our backs. In other words, we're focused on the impossible task of making our bodies (or our weddings or our cars or our children) perfect. The point is, instead of looking at the real problems facing us as a country, as a culture, and as citizens of the world, we have tried to make the everyday surfaces of our lives shiny and bright, like plastic. And it's time to think about how we got here and what we're going to do now. This book is about Americans and our ability to reshape ourselves and our money into an infinite variety of new forms. It's also about our ability to stop. There is a breaking point of any material, even plastic. We have reached that breaking point.

In this endpoint of our plastic time and place, plastic surgeons have successfully performed face transplants, and ordinary shoppers can wander into walk-in Botox clinics. No appointment necessary to have a neurotoxin that causes botulism injected into our faces, thereby freezing time and all facial expression. The simultaneous existence of face transplants and voluntary facial paralysis surely signals that we are at an interesting historical juncture. Our older notions of self and body are being replaced by more postmodern realities. Now our desires and our bodies can intersect with technology and finance to form a seamless whole. Our very American belief that we can always improve ourselves, as well as the equally American belief that our bodies require work, has melted into a technologically advanced and profit-driven plastic surgery industry.

I use the term "plastic surgery" throughout this book. Like most Americans, when I refer to plastic surgery, I don't mean reconstructive surgery, but cosmetic surgery. This is something that drives plastic surgeon friends crazy. "There's a big difference between giving a woman breast implants after she's had a double mastectomy and giving big boobs to a skinny teenager" scolds one. I know. I agree, mostly. Reconstructive surgery, the sort of surgery that is done after an accident or disease or because of birth anomalies, is not the same as cosmetic surgery.

On the other hand, an editor of a women's magazine once told me that there is no line at all. "Most cosmetic surgery is actually reconstructive," she insisted. "If you think of how difficult it is to go around in a body that isn't attractive, then there's no difference between getting liposuction or a nose job and getting your face reconstructed after a car accident." I want to disagree, but the line between "necessary" and "unnecessary" is not exactly clear. Consider bariatric surgery, or stomach stapling, as it is commonly known. Bariatric surgery is for the extremely obese. Is stomach stapling cosmetic or reconstructive given that the patient could, in theory, lose the weight through diet and exercise? What about after losing three hundred pounds, when the patient's stomach skin now sags past his knees? Is the skin-tightening surgery afterwards necessary?

I am going to pretend the line is there, even if it is constantly being erased. Cosmetic surgery is unnecessary; reconstructive surgery is sometimes necessary for the patient and sometimes necessary for the average-bodied people who have to live with the patient. In this book, I'm talking about the unnecessary kind of surgery—breast implants or smaller noses or thinner midsections or fewer wrinkles. In this book, plastic surgery is done to change the surfaces of our bodies. It has nothing to do with health. Of course, sometimes reconstructive surgery has nothing to do with health. Sometimes it's just about our unease with bodies that are different. Humans have always been both attracted to and repulsed by those who are bodily "freaks." No doubt this is where the impulse for plastic surgery in its reconstructive sense came from: an impulse to make freaks disappear. But despite what might be a deep human impulse to look at or look away from bodily difference, it was only in the 1890s that people began to consider voluntarily going under the knife. Cosmetic surgery became an industry, and once people with more or less "normal" and "functional" bodies could pay to have themselves reshaped, there was no turning back. Plastic surgery went from fixing what was "wrong" with people to "correcting" difference, and it did so at a nice profit.

This book explores the explosion of cosmetic surgery in the last twenty years, as it went from a way for the elite to "normalize" their looks to a much more widespread standardization of Americans' bodies and faces. In order to understand this transformation, we have to understand not just plastic surgery but plastic money. In this book, I rely on a lot of other people's work on the American economy and debt and the beauty and plastic surgery industries, but I also use years of my own fieldwork. I have interviewed over a hundred patients and plastic surgeons from all over the world, watched hundreds of hours of plastic surgery television shows, and even systematically read women's magazines for advertisements and articles on plastic surgery.

In the first section, "American Plastic," I look at plastic surgery in its powerful and yet culturally specific form in the United States. Chapter 1, "A Short History of Plastic," provides background on the technological and cultural forces that gave birth to cosmetic surgery. Chapter 2, "The State of Plastic," looks at how a political revolution in the United States in the 1980s created the perfect state for the explosion of cosmetic surgery and debt. Chapter 3, "Plastic People and Their Doctors," looks at plastic surgery as an industry and at the people who are its practitioners and customers. It is based on my interviews with plastic surgeons and their patients over the course of the past several years.

The second section, "Boob Jobs and Credit Cards," asks, "Why do we Americans want plastic surgery?" and "How will we pay for it?" In Chapter 4, "Learning to Be Plastic," I look at how the desire for cosmetic surgery is implanted through cultural scripts such as women's magazines and TV shows. These scripts encourage us, or at least some of us, to get cosmetic surgery. In Chapter 5, "The Mirror and the Porn Star," I look at how the increasing availability of pornography as well as the increasingly surgically altered body of the porn star can create a desire for cosmetic surgery. Chapter 6, "Broken Plastic," explores what happened to plastic surgery after the plastic money dried up.

The third and final section is "The Quest for Perfection." Chapter 7, "Resistance," considers how "perfection" may contain the seeds of its own destruction by demanding so much from us that we eventually rise up and resist. The concluding chapter, ". . . Is Futile?" is my attempt to put to rest once and for all the claim that plastic surgery is inevitable. A large number of experts, from evolutionary biologists to TV personalities, tell us that we cannot avoid cosmetic surgery, because "youth" and "beauty" are hardwired into us, and body work is required in order for us to get ahead. Conservative politicians and pundits tell us that greed need not be regulated. But humans create our realities, and none of these realities are predetermined or inevitable. Cultural scripts are not written in stone, but in performance. Humans might perform plastic differently in the future than we do now. Some of us are already doing so. All of these chapters will, in the end, show what we knew from the beginning: that there's one word we should be listening to. That word is "plastic."

PART I

American Plastic

CHAPTER 1

A Short History of Plastic

Make It Go Away

Sitting in a colleague's office, discussing my work, we move from MTV's *I Want a Famous Face,* a reality-TV show where young people undergo a series of surgical procedures to look like Brad Pitt or J-Lo, to face transplants—once a rare and heroic surgery that is quickly becoming commonplace.[1] We laugh about living in "interesting times," the curse that surely signals this moment, when wanting Brad Pitt's face and actually having Brad Pitt's face are both possibilities. I am startled to hear him announce: "You're against cosmetic surgery."

Against cosmetic surgery? That's like being against the automobile: a possibly ethical stance, but nonetheless impossible, or at least highly impractical, especially if you live in a place without any public transportation or, in the case of plastic surgery, a body that's aging. Ever since I started researching this subject, people have pointedly asked me what I think of cosmetic surgery, as if my opinion matters, like if I say, "It's a bad thing," it will go away. Or perhaps some hope I'll respond, "It's a good thing," and validate their secret desire to get work done. The truth is simply this: the historical, cultural, and economic forces that brought us to this point are so strong, the roots of our obsession with cosmetic surgery run so deep into the very essence of what it means to be an American, that there is no escape. Still, perhaps understanding how we got here, the history of this moment, will in fact allow us to think about alternative paths. Even if knowing the history of cosmetic surgery doesn't free us from its grip, it's a hell of a story.

The kind of story you can't make up, because it's just too crazy to be anything but true.

Some historians start the tale of cosmetic surgery in ancient India, sometime around 600 BCE. Apparently a common punishment for adultery was cutting off the adulterer's nose. And so there were a lot of people running around without noses. The surgeons attempted to make something that resembled a nose by cutting a flap of skin from the forehead and grafting it onto the face where the nose should have been. This was of course done without the benefit of anesthesia, but then again, so was cutting off their noses in the first place.[2] In Renaissance Italy, surgeons began to speak of "aesthetic" or "beauty" surgery, but they meant procedures like reconstructing the nose after it had collapsed due to syphilis.[3]

Surgery to put a nose back on the face is more reconstructive than aesthetic in nature. Surgery to reshape the "normal" body, surgery for purely cosmetic reasons, only began at the end of the 1800s. The sort of cosmetic surgery practices that are flourishing in the twenty-first century are about standardizing bodies, not reconstructing them after disfiguring accidents or disease. As philosopher and historian Michel Foucault put it, there are a variety of modern institutions and practices that act as if "they are intended to alleviate pain, to cure, to comfort, but which all tend . . . to exercise a power of normalization."[4] Purely cosmetic surgery is a thoroughly modern phenomenon, the purpose of which is the normalization of bodies.

Before modernity, a body that was different was always more powerful and often more dangerous than an average body. Freakish bodies required explanation. A cleft palate might be punishment for gossiping. Conjoined twins might signal good luck for an entire village. The anomalous body was interpreted as a sign of divine wrath or divine grace, but the freakish body was never ignored. As evolutionary biologist Armand Marie Leroi tells us, in *Mutants,* "In the sixteenth and seventeenth centuries, monsters were everywhere. Princes collected them; naturalists catalogued them; theologians turned them into religious propaganda."[5] At some point, the impulse to interpret the anomalous body, to make the freak mean something, transformed into an impulse to reshape that body and ultimately make the freak disappear from view. It is at this moment, as those with anomalous bodies moved from a sign from God to a source of disgust, that cosmetic surgery is born. As disability studies scholar Rosemarie Garland Thomson explains it, "what was once sought after as revelation . . . now inspires horror; what was taken as a portent shifts to a site of progress. In brief, wonder becomes error."[6] This desire to normalize freakish bodies is at the very center of what it means to be modern.

A century ago, crowds gathered at freak shows to gawk and stare and pay a dime to see the wondrous diversity of the human form. A century before that, they gathered in front of churches and in marketplaces to hear priests tell them to look at divinity in the limits of the human flesh. By the 1930s, the new religions of science and "beauty capitalism"—markets that both implant the need to transform our ordinary into something more beautiful and extract profit from that need—worked together to signal freaks as a failure. This moment of turning away from abnormal bodies is perfectly captured in the opening sequence of the 1932 Tod Browning horror film *Freaks*. The movie features some of the biggest stars of the freak show, people like Daisy and Violet Hilton, conjoined twins who starred on Broadway and in film, and Johnny Eck, a man born without his lower half and known as the Human Torso. As the lengthy prologue scrolls across the screen, the following line jumps out as both the dream and the nightmare of the thoroughly modern desire for normalization: "Never again will such a story be filmed, as modern science and teratology is rapidly eliminating such blunders of nature from the world." Browning's film caused shock and disgust among its contemporary viewers. The film was quickly removed from circulation. By 1932, such extreme bodily diversity was too horrible to watch.[7]

The impulse to normalize freakish bodies, to make them disappear, is something that developed over time. It required the creation of certain ideologies, especially racial ideologies like eugenics, as well as certain technologies, like instrument sterilization. Cosmetic surgery also required the development of a visual culture, the large-scale urbanization and migration that meant people were increasingly judged on appearances, and a consumer capitalism that sold beauty as a form of self-improvement.

As freakish bodies became increasingly reshaped, other bodies came under scrutiny: the fat, the aging, the not fully white. The modern body must look as if it is productive and "healthy," but it must also look like it belongs to the dominant racial and economic groups, which is another way of saying "beautiful." Modernity demanded that not just the living but also the dead be made to look both "beautiful" and "healthy." Part of the story of cosmetic surgery is that it developed alongside the funeral industry. In the same way that technological developments worked with beauty capitalism to create cosmetic surgery, embalming techniques and entrepreneurs of death transformed the corpse into a body that looked "good."[8] Sometime around 1880, the modern body, dead or alive, started to require the services of experts. Since then, more and more of us feel the need to go under the knife in this life and get embalmed for the next.

The Technology of Cosmetic Surgery

When I interview cosmetic surgeons, they often describe the history of their field as one of military service, of hero-surgeons piecing back the broken bodies of soldiers during war. A 1948 *Atlas of Cosmetic Surgery* is typical of this:

The past thirty years, during which two World Wars were fought, have been the most momentous—indeed without parallel—in the evolution of plastic surgery as an art and a science. The lay public . . . has of late years become cognizant of the truly amazing results often obtained through plastic surgery—results not only of purely esthetic and functional nature but of definite value psychologically, socially, and economically.[9]

Many historians of plastic surgery agree that it was the wars, particularly World War I, that gave birth to plastic surgery. World War I was fought in trenches, with soldiers' bodies more or less protected but their heads vulnerable to enemy attack. Trench warfare resulted in an unprecedented number of facial injuries that could not be hidden from view except through surgery.[10] Often, cosmetic surgery is traced even farther back, to the horribly disfigured bodies left in the wake of the American Civil War. The sort of ammunition introduced during this war was much more likely to wound the face, and surgeons became increasingly skilled at rebuilding the facial structure.[11]

No doubt war increased the technical skills of reconstructive surgeons dramatically. But the real technological breakthroughs for cosmetic surgery were figuring out how to anesthetize a patient, and also how to sterilize instruments so that chances of survival after the operation increased dramatically. In other words, plastic surgery had to become less painful and less fatal to attract its actual audience: *the normal*. Soldiers from any war who were left with crumpled faces were willing to take their chances; but someone with a big nose or a sagging jaw line was not going to go under the knife fully awake and likely to get sepsis and die. Or as Ralph Waldo Emerson once observed, and the true believers in the magic of capitalism often quote: "Build a better mouse trap and the world will beat a path to your door."

So it is that aesthetic surgery shifted from reconstructive to cosmetic, and the recipients of such surgeries moved from being patients to being consumers. Of course, what trapped us, what made us keep coming back for more and more, was the irresistible mix of beauty and bodily transcendence that cosmetic surgery promised.

Consuming Beauty

It is difficult to imagine a world where beauty is not a product. After more than a hundred years of shopping for beauty, how can we imagine that it once existed outside of the market? Seeing beauty as something to be bought is part of a larger revolution that took place alongside industrialization and capitalism. That revolution was all about shopping, shopping for beauty and for our selves. At the same time cosmetic surgery was born, so was the department store. Both signaled a change in how we Americans defined ourselves and our happiness. We were no longer producers, but consumers. And we were only successful to the extent that we could consume more this year than last, more next year than this. Through shopping we learned to construct ourselves and our relationship to others. And it was middle-class white women who were first released from production in order to go on shopping sprees. That's why the first shopping areas were called Ladies' Mile. These ladies no longer made things like soap or clothes in the home; instead they entered department stores, palaces of desire, and started the revolution now known as consumer capitalism.[12] At the center of ladies' shopping was the desire for a newly created product: "beauty."

This moment of some women shifting their roles from producer to consumer and moving from the domestic realm into the newly invented public spaces of shopping is extremely important to the history of cosmetic surgery and, no doubt, the world more generally. Shopping for beauty was not completely dominated by profit alone. There was always an incredible optimism, and even a democratic spirit, to the beauty industry. For the first time in human history beauty wasn't something one was born with, a sort of luck of the genetic draw, but something one worked at with the aid of a variety of products, from slimming corsets to rouge to, at least by the twentieth century, cosmetic surgery. Buying beauty was an all-American activity.[13]

There were a variety of forces at play on the American lady consumer, not least of which was a new form of communication: advertising. The first advertisements were for items previously made in the home, things like soap and sewing machines. Feminist scholar Anne McClintock sees early advertisements as a form of "commodity racism." In other words, ladies bought into advertising not just to make themselves better, more like the people in the ads, but also to make themselves safe. Products like soap promised to protect consumers from becoming infected with the "dirt" of other races or classes. The modern city brought a lot of confusion and boundary crossing, especially in the lives of "lady shoppers."[14]

In the same way that soap advertised protection from social "dirt," the beauty industry promised to protect ladies from ugliness. Beauty products provided boundary protection between the revolting and ugly working woman and the clean and beautiful lady of leisure. Beauty products protected middle-class white ladies from class and race contamination, and they simultaneously offered the promise of redemption for working women to become more "beautiful" and therefore "ladylike." Consider the text from a 1934 advertisement for Camay soap.

> Beauty-beauty-beauty! Life's a constant search for it . . . For wherever you go, someone's eyes appraise you, someone's mind is made up—a friendship or an aversion is formed. You cannot, of course, change the contour of your chin or the color of your eyes. But you can change . . . the condition of your skin.[15]

With cosmetic surgery and other forms of plastic beauty, people could and would change the contour of their chin, the shape of their noses, even the color of their skin, not just to be more beautiful, but to resemble those with the most money and power; that is, to be more white.

Cosmetic Surgery and Race

The heart of the matter in aesthetic surgery is the common human desire to "pass."

—SANDER L. GILMAN

It was not just beauty that trapped Americans in the culture of cosmetic surgery—it was race. Early cosmetic surgery consumers were lured by the promise of a body free from the racial features that marked them as degenerate. Within the racial science of the time, certain genetic pathologies were clearly visible on the body. Scientists could see criminality in the slope of a forehead. Primitive, atavistic natures were marked by the width of the nose, even the fleshiness of the ears. This obsession with racial superiority and bodily differences began long before cosmetic surgery became a viable commercial industry. In 1812 crowds in London couldn't stop staring at the shockingly "degenerate" body of the Hottentot Venus, a young Khoisan woman by the name of Saartje Baartman whose "protruding labia" and large buttocks caused a frenzy of looking among the respectable classes. These supposedly obvious signs of African degeneracy were caught up in efforts to justify the British Empire and the racial hierarchies that privileged European over African.[16] A century later, a display in the chimpanzee cage at the Bronx Zoo of a young Bachichiri (Pygmy) man by the name of Ota Benga caused a similar frenzy of looking and seeing racial degeneracy in everything from Benga's teeth to his stature. Grappling with the effects of segregation and white supremacy, Americans rushed to the zoo to stare at the nearly naked and clearly "primitive" body of Mr. Benga.[17] Imagine the fear that those with the bodily features of degeneracy must have felt. At any moment, you could be put on display as a freak, an animal, a scientific exhibit showing the superiority of whiteness.

Erasing degeneracy and difference has long been the project of cosmetic surgery. From the late 1800s on, cosmetic surgery was always about making the not yet fully white able to pass. Racial hierarchies "create an ideal arena for aesthetic surgery, with its promise to help people 'pass' as whoever they wish to be."[18] Almost as soon as surgeons figured out how to put their patients out with gas, they began to sell surgery as the cure for Jewish and Irish noses, that is, the cure for being marked as racially "other." In Japan, where aesthetic surgery appeared about the same time as the introduction of Western medicine in the late 1800s, eyelids were quickly "fixed" with a double fold.[19] Race and empire melted together with cosmetic surgery to produce technologies that loosened the body from racial markers, thereby fixing whiteness as that which is to be desired and purchased. Furthermore, making the body more "beautiful" increasingly came to be seen as a cure for unhappiness.[20]

And what was this unhappiness of the psyche that cosmetic surgery promised to cure? It was, of course, an unhappiness with the stigmata of race.[21] Because much of American life due to slavery, and European life due to empire, was predicated on a racial hierarchy, having racial difference written on the body marked the body as diseased and inferior. Cosmetic surgery "tried to correct the 'ugliness' of nonwhite races . . . Racial science used appearance as a means of determining who was fit and who was ill, who could reproduce and 'improve' the race and who should be excluded and condemned."[22] The connection between "beauty surgery" and eugenics was there from the beginning.

Eugenics, like the physical-fitness movement of the early twentieth century, envisioned modernity as creating physical decay, a decay that was a threat to the nation. The response in the

United States was mass sterilization of "imbeciles" and the "unfit," as well as family-planning campaigns, sports, and an effort to strengthen the nation one individual at a time. By the time Adolf Hitler adopted eugenics for his own Final Solution, it was already an internationally accepted scientific belief, *and* a popular one. But in America, especially by the 1930s, eugenicists were embracing both a hereditary model (genes) and an environmental one (improve yourself). In perhaps a uniquely American way, with the emphasis on the possibility of success through hard work, eugenics became not just about birth, but also about lifestyle. Eugenics American-style worked for the reproduction of the perfect baby, but also to convince adults to adopt new regimes of fitness, health, *and* beauty.[23] Indeed, it made total sense for a famous eugenicist like Albert E. Wiggam to judge the 1929 Miss Universe pageant, since beauty was both a sign of genetic superiority and something we have to work at.[24] And if you couldn't work away the signs of genetic inferiority, then cosmetic surgeons could. Beauty surgery, not a soap or a cream, was the only product that could truly protect us from ugliness.

Cosmetic surgery as a commercial enterprise embedded in racial hierarchies continued to expand throughout the twentieth century. Until the 1970s, more than half of all rhinoplasty patients in the United States were Jews. The Jewish nose, hypervisible as a sign of racial difference, was easily transformed, thereby allowing Jews to become fully "white," at least in the United States. As Virginia Blum says in *Flesh Wounds,* her semiautobiographical account of cosmetic surgery: "The story of my household is like that of many Jewish American families whose assimilation is symbolized through physical appearance . . . Certain kinds of noses speak Jewishness. Jews assimilating into a largely gentile culture thus strip from our features traces of our ethnicity."[25]

Africans on display like Baartman and Benga had little chance of using cosmetic surgery to "pass" as evolved creatures, but other groups, like Jews and Irish and even African Americans, quickly realized that what the industry of cosmetic surgery could give them was an escape from their racially degenerate bodies. Much of the earliest commercial cosmetic surgeries were more about passing as "healthy" and escaping the "diseased" racially other body than about "beauty."[26]

Passing as white was the raison d'être for cosmetic surgery as an industry; but cosmetic surgery was particularly interested in the "beauty" of white women. This is why it quickly went from an industry primarily concerned with Jewish and Irish men to one almost exclusively concerned with women. It's not that race went away as the central concern of cosmetic surgery; it's that racial purity was marked almost exclusively on the bodies of women. Within the racial science of the time, degeneracy was most often marked as a lack of gender differentiation. Scientific racism interpreted those cultures and races and classes that did not have highly feminine women and highly masculine men as degenerate, and the white middle class, with its working men and domestic ladies, as highly evolved.

That's how cosmetic surgery's racial project of helping people look whiter also became a highly gendered project of helping women look more feminine. Sexologist Havelock Ellis wrote more than a century ago that "the question of sex—with the racial questions that rest on it—stands before the coming generations as the chief problem for solution."[27] The question of sex and the racial problem were always one and the same. Any deviation from gender or class norms—union activism, homosexuality, prostitution—was considered a form of racial degeneracy.[28] In other words, a body that was not clearly gendered as masculine or feminine presented a threat to the racial and class order. Fixing signs of imperfect masculinity or femininity became a way of moving up the race-class hierarchy, a way of becoming not only whiter, but also having more "class." So it is that the racial project of passing got permanently entangled with the feminine task of beauty.

But cosmetic surgery didn't just get entangled in race, it got entangled in celebrity. By the 1870s, newspapers began to advertise a variety of beauty products. The number of products "respectable" women could consume, including cosmetics, increased over time. Perhaps more importantly, celebrities began to endorse beauty products, thus instilling a desire in the women buying them to look like the celebrity, or at least like her photograph. Celebrity culture, beauty products, and advertising all arose alongside cosmetic surgery as an industry. Women consumers were trapped in a matrix of the unattainable celebrity beauty and the enticing promises of advertising.[29]

Prestigious Imitation

In 1891 the Edison Company showed what might have been the first film on its patented new machine, the kinetoscope. Within a few years, the motion picture industry was born. The filmic age changed the way we viewed ourselves because it changed what we wanted to be. Anthropologists tell us that in all societies, humans imitate those with the most prestige, a process called "prestigious imitation." This may seem obvious until we think about how radically prestige changed with the twin birth of photography and advertising. Previously we might have looked to our parents or older siblings, village elders, or even the queen as the most prestigious and therefore worthy of imitation, but with the invention of cinema and the creation of movie stars, all that changed.

Early on in the cinematic era, anthropologist Marcel Mauss understood we were starting to shape our very bodies in an effort to imitate matinee idols. Writing in 1934, Mauss had a "revelation" while lying in a hospital bed in New York.

I wondered where previously I had seen girls walking as my nurses walked. I had the time to think about it. At last I realized that it was at the cinema. Returning to France, I noticed how common this gait was, especially in Paris; the girls were French and they too were walking in this way. In fact, American walking fashions had begun to arrive over here, thanks to the cinema.[30]

More recently, philosopher Jean Baudrillard pointed out that it is not the actual people, but rather representations of people, copies without an original, that we imitate when we try to become like movie stars.[31] In other words, I may want to look like Jennifer Lopez, but chances are that I will never see the actual Jennifer Lopez, and if I did, I probably wouldn't recognize her. What I want to be is like the images of J-Lo that saturate our culture and my imagination.

Thus, the fact that photography, advertising, and cosmetic surgery became industries at the same time is not a historical accident, but a causal equation.[32] What the age of photography did to prestigious imitation was to condense it to a moment frozen in time and two-dimensional space. Looking good now requires that we make dynamic, three-dimensional bodies more like photographs, imitations of an imitation, so that we all become reproductions without an original. But even the originals, the movie stars themselves, had to increasingly get cosmetic surgery to look "good" on film.

Cosmetic Surgery and Sex

By the 1920s, Americans were obsessed with the actress Fanny Brice's nose job. The mixture of sex and race in Brice's career is impossible to fully separate, since it was her Jewish*ness* that made her "funny" (as immortalized by Barbra Streisand in *Funny Girl*), but it was the fact that Brice wanted to look "beautiful"—which is to say fully female and white—that made her undergo a nose job in 1923.[33] Since then, the bodies that we want to imitate are not just two-dimensional and therefore unreal, but surgically altered before they're even photographed. We now imitate bodies that never existed. Through

prestigious imitation, plastic surgery has spread from being a
necessity for matinee idols to a necessity for the rest of us, as
we are all trapped in a two-dimensional visual culture that rewards bodies that look good on-screen. Because women were
the first shoppers and continue to dominate consumption, ac-
counting for about 80 percent of all purchases, they were also
the most obvious audience for advertisers.[34] Advertising taught
women—and then men—to want to look like bodies that cannot exist "in nature."

So it was that being a woman in the twentieth century often required not just cosmetics, but cosmetic surgery. Both the
first professional meeting of plastic surgeons and the first Miss
America pageant were held in the late summer of 1921 because
both wanted the same thing: clearly gendered, classed and raced
beauties.[35] The obsession with the female body continued to
dominate cosmetic surgery throughout the century. The Depression came and went, but it did nothing to slow the growth
of the cosmetics industry aimed almost exclusively at women.[36]
Cosmetic surgery continued to spread, reaching the upper middle classes in addition to the rich and famous.

World War II left a longing for large breasts in its wake,
a longing that fed a growing practice in breast augmentation.
Why Americans suddenly became obsessed with large breasts is
an interesting question. Some theorize that it was the depriva-
tion of the two wars and the Depression that caused a desire for
women who looked full and abundant. Others theorize that it
was the "foundation garment" industry that first invented the bra
in the 1930s, with its cup sizes that required all women to fit into
them or feel like a misfit. Surely 1950s anxiety over producing a
"normal" girl, which increasingly fed into young girls' desires for
large breasts, shaped this obsession with "the sweater girl."[37]

The year 1959 proved to be a watershed year for cosmetic
surgery, since that was when Barbie was introduced to the
American toy market and an entire generation of young girls

grew up worshiping a form impossible to achieve without surgical intervention. As M. G. Lord points out in her biography
of Barbie:

> In Barbie's early years, Mattel struggled to make its doll
> look like a real-life movie star. Today, however, real-life ce-
> lebrities—as well as common folk—are emulating her. The
> postsurgical Dolly Parton looks like the postsurgical Ivana
> Trump looks like the postsurgical Michael Jackson looks
> like the postsurgical Joan Rivers looks like . . . Barbie."[38]

Women and even young girls became increasingly obsessed
with having large breasts. "We must, we must, we must improve our busts" was chanted over and over again as a fervent
prayer for C cups. Psychiatry named distress over small breasts
"a significant problem."[39] Popular magazines and beauty advice
books also "worried" about the size of women's breasts.[40] A variety of advertisements and articles offered breasts as a means
of escaping the confinement of women's postwar roles. For instance, the Maidenform "I Dream . . ." campaign, introduced
in 1949, was the first advertising campaign to feature a woman
in her underwear. The ads had women "dream" they went to
Paris or won a political election or even just went shopping in
their Maidenform bras. The Maidenform "Dream" campaign is
"a classic example of wish-fulfillment psychology, as the fantasy
situations of the ads fed women's hunger for independence, romance, personal achievement, and even power and influence."[41]
Ever anxious to please the public, plastic surgeons began
experimenting with breast augmentation. Earlier surgeons had
tried paraffin and fat injections, but the results were not good,
and often deadly. In the early 1950s plastic surgeons tried med-
ical-grade sponge implants. The sponges made the breasts look
a bit like the padded bras that were also popular. The sponges
didn't really work, since they tended to harden and were often

impossible to remove because surrounding tissue usually filled in and embedded the porous sponges. Increasingly, doctors and patients turned to silicone injections directly into the breasts, a highly dangerous practice that was allowed to continue for decades. By the early 1960s, the silicone implant had been invented, as well as early attempts at saline sacs that could be filled to capacity once inside the woman's breasts. Although hardly perfect—for instance, the ridges usually could be felt through the skin—these implants were more or less stable, possibly safe, and, unlike earlier implants, did not result in disfigurement and scarring if they needed to be removed.[42]

Saline and silicone implants, however, were not the final solution for big breasts, since many women claimed that the implants made them sick. In response to complaints about their safety, silicone implants were removed from the American market in 1992. In the rest of the world, silicone remained the implant of choice. After decades of lawsuits and scientific studies, the expert consensus was that silicone implants are safe, and so they were reintroduced in 2006.[43] Legal or not, there remains a large disconnect between the experiences of many women who received breast implants and the plastic surgeons who put them in. Again and again, the doctors who do implants insist that they are "perfectly safe," while many women say their boob jobs made them sick. As Beauty and the Breast, a blog started by activists against silicone implants, insists, "breast implants are not safe, yet demand for this invasive cosmetic surgery continues to skyrocket. The reasons for this are many, varied and complex, involving fundamental questions about the meaning of beauty, self worth and the role of women in a supposedly enlightened 21st century society."[44] At Implants Out, Kacey Long rails against the supposedly safer saline implants. According to Long, her implants sickened her with rheumatoid arthritis, and only after their removal did she start to recover.[45]

Whatever the truth about the safety of implants, breasts

have remained at the center of both cosmetic surgery and feminine beauty for decades. Thus it is not surprising that when
feminist activists gathered in September of 1968 to protest the
Miss America pageant in Atlantic City, they chose to burn their
bras and call the contest a "degrading mindless-boob-girlie symbol."[46] In mid-century America, the bra, more than the implant,
represented the oppression of women. With their padded and
canonical shapes that forced breasts to stand erect, bras represented exactly how women's bodies could no longer be beautiful
without external intervention. Besides, it was probably easier to
burn bras than breast implants.

Despite the feminist backlash against the beauty industry,
cosmetic surgery continued to flourish, at least for certain women
and a few men. As feminism and its bra-burning righteousness
came and went over the next couple of decades, cosmetic surgery
became even more popular as it managed to reinvent itself as
"empowering to women." Cosmetic surgeons urged women to
exercise their right to a "choice," and assured them that investment in cosmetic procedures was a necessary step to career success. Plastic surgeons were advertising both breast implants and
liposuction as a career investment.[47] During these years, wom-
en's labor-force participation increased dramatically from about
one-third to slightly under half of all workers.[48] An investment
in one's career through one's body made perfect sense.

By 1981, when Nancy Reagan, with her surgically enhanced
face, became First Lady,[49] plastic surgery was the fastest-growing subspecialty in American medicine.[50] In 1982 plastic surgeons and other medical professionals were allowed to advertise
for the first time under new, federally enforced guidelines for
the American Medical Association.[51] The advertisements for
cosmetic surgeons quickly became the most numerous and, like
all advertising, were not necessarily the best way for patients to
get the information they needed.

Along with the deregulation of medical advertising, the

Reagan years brought the introduction of liposuction to the American market. Despite some initial problems, like death due to pulmonary embolisms, it quickly became one of the most popular surgical procedures in the United States.[52] In yet another ironic twist of fate that indicates the gods may be plastic surgeons, Americans began to get fatter. From 1980 to 2000, obesity rates doubled.[53] By 1988, about 1.5 million Americans purchased some sort of cosmetic surgery, with breast implants and liposuction being the most popular procedures. And the people getting cosmetic surgery, mostly women, were not necessarily the rich and famous, one survey showing that nearly half of them earned less than $25,000 a year.[54]

In 1997 over 2 million Americans were going to a board-certified cosmetic surgeon for surgical and nonsurgical procedures. This actually means that more Americans were getting "work" done, since any medical practitioner is allowed to perform cosmetic procedures, but the only data available is through professional groups like the American Society for Aesthetic Plastic Surgery (ASAPS). Interestingly, nearly 14 percent of cosmetic surgery patients were men. The most common surgical procedure for Americans was liposuction, with eyelid lifts and boob jobs not far behind. Just two years later, in 1999, that number rose to 4.6 million Americans visiting a board-certified plastic surgeon. About 11 percent of the patients were men and the most popular procedures were liposuction and breast augmentation.

This pattern of plastic beauty luring more and more Americans to the plastic surgeon's office continued, despite economic downturns and terrorist attacks. In 2000 there were 5.7 million cosmetic procedures, a 173 percent increase in three years. Men still accounted for 11 percent of the patients. In 2001 Americans had 8.5 million cosmetic procedures. This number dropped slightly in 2002, to 6.9 million, no doubt due to the national trauma of 9/11, but quickly climbed to nearly 12 million by 2004, and then dropped slightly to 10.2 million in 2008. In

2008 the drop was probably related to the economic recession, but can also be explained by the increasing number of patients who go outside the United States or just outside of board-certified surgeons for the cheapest possible procedures. Also, cosmetic treatments like Botox are increasingly performed not by surgeons, but by aestheticians and other beauty purveyors.[55]

The real big news in 2008 was that breast implants beat out liposuction as the most popular procedure. That's because nearly 90 percent of cosmetic surgery patients were women after 2007. Why women mostly wanted boob jobs is not clear. Alan Gold, the president of ASAPS, theorizes that it has to do with changing fashions: "For the first time in the twelve years these statistics have been collected liposuction is a runner up in popularity to breast augmentation. [This reflects] changes in fashion, i.e. décolletage baring styles, might be a factor behind this change."[56]

Yes, perhaps, but it may have more to do with the role of women during economic downturns. This "lipstick effect" was first noted by Leonard Lauder, of Estée Lauder, who saw lipstick sales jump after 9/11 and theorized that in tough times, people need "small luxuries."[57] But why is it that women buy lipstick and boob jobs and men buy ties? Perhaps it is because men must look as if they're doing well economically, even when they're not, whereas women's economic well-being is caught up in being beautiful. Or, as Simone de Beauvoir told us in *The Second Sex,* "the toilette is not only adornment . . . it also indicates woman's social situation."[58]

Finding Meaning in Plastic Beauty

Why this expansion of beauty regimes in the 1980s? And why was it mostly white women who consumed cosmetic surgery? A variety of scholars tried to figure out the meaning of the expansion of the cosmetic surgery industry in spite of, or even perhaps because of, feminism. Susan Faludi famously argued that the beauty industry, which includes cosmetic surgery, was part of a

larger backlash against the gains women had made in the 1970s
and 1980s. According to Faludi, the more progress women make
in their careers, the more they must be punished with, among
other things, an ever-increasing need to work for beauty.[59] Few
beauty regimens require more work than going under the knife.
A similar argument was taken up by Naomi Wolf in *The Beauty
Myth*, again positing that the beauty industry imbues women
with "needs" that can only be satisfied through endless consumption of products, including cosmetic surgery.[60]

These feminist accounts have initiated a decade of disavowals
from other scholars who argue that making women "victims" of
the cosmetic surgery industry is not only disempowering, but also
doesn't account for the real-life pleasures and satisfactions women
get from pursuing beauty. Kathy Davis, in *Reshaping the Female
Body*, was one of the first to argue that women are getting cosmetic
surgery not because they're dupes of the beauty industry, but because it is a rational way of negotiating social power. Davis's book
is based on sociological research in the Netherlands, a place where
cosmetic surgery was often paid for by the national health service.
Under these conditions, outside of the high costs and high debt
that are the price of plastic beauty in most countries, Davis can
argue that getting cosmetic surgery can be described as a rational
decision. Davis urges us to "find ways to explore cosmetic surgery
as a complex and dilemmatic situation for women: problem and
solution, oppression and liberation, all in one."[61] In other words,
given that women who are closer to the standards of beauty really will be treated better at work and at home, it is a perfectly
reasonable choice to reshape the body to be more like the standard. In *Amending the Abject Body*, Deborah Coslav Covino agrees
with Davis that going under the knife can be a "self-conscious and
well-informed decision," and one taken in an effort to reconcile
our sense of self with the abjection of our bodies that is so central
to our culture.[62]

Still other scholars see cosmetic surgery as part of a larger "body project." This obsession with the body as a potentially perfectible entity became central to American culture sometime in the 1970s with the introduction of "exercise culture" for women and men of all ages. As Debra Gimlin points out,

Nearly four decades after the beginning of the most recent fitness craze, the popularity of body work shows few signs of letting up. Throughout the United States, women are lifting weights to build muscle; wrapping their bodies in seaweed to reduce water retention; jogging on athletic tracks, highways, and mountain trails; attending weekly weigh-ins at their local diet centers; and participating in any number of other activities intended to alter the appearance of their bodies.[63]

In this sense, cosmetic surgery is just part of a larger project of making ourselves "better" by changing the way we look.

More recent scholarship has focused on how cosmetic surgery is situated in a larger global economy that has displaced many of us and made nearly all of us more insecure about our futures. In a world culture where the body is treated as a commodity, we have no choice but to "invest" in its beauty and therefore its marketability. In *Making the Cut,* Anthony Elliot argues that cosmetic surgery is a direct result of globalization. Our newfound obsession with creating the perfect body is the result of the radical insecurity we now have at work and at home. Our very tenuous position in the economy and society is what makes "cosmetic surgical culture . . . one of excess, fear, disposability, anxieties, and melancholia . . . The culture of spectacle and short-termism promoted by the global electronic economy . . . introduces fundamental anxieties and insecurities that are increasingly resolved by individuals at the level of the body."[64]

Interesting Times

Elliot is right. The explosion of plastic surgery is a direct result of the global economy. Gilman is right that the large presence of plastic in our cultural landscape is a new form of eugenics, a reinvigorated obsession with the body as an indicator of our core character as well as a variety of technological innovation. I also have no doubt that earlier feminist critiques of the cosmetic surgery industry, like Wolf's, were correct. There is a pattern of fear and loathing when it comes to certain bodies in our culture. For white, aging women, that fear and loathing is played out through the need for cosmetic intervention. It plays out differently for Black women or gay men or whatever other bodies we love to hate. Plastic beauty is a feminist issue as well as a racial and financial one. And, like Davis, I would argue that the consumers of cosmetic beauty are doing the best they can in circumstances not of their own making. The story of cosmetic surgery really is not that different from the story of the automobile. We might prefer to not go under the knife, but what choice do we have? To be ugly? And how will that get us anywhere? Pretending that you don't have to get in the car, or get the Botox, or dye your gray hair in order to thrive is more a sign of being extremely out of touch with reality than of empowerment.

But there's something else afoot, something that is not universal, but particular. Plastic is central to who we are as Americans. Plastic money is at the center of all of this. America pioneered plastic money, and Americans led the world in their willingness to use plastic money—debt—to finance the present. This willingness to "take risks" with plastic money is rooted in what economists like to call Americans' "optimism bias." Americans, more than other people, tend to assume that the future will always be better. Also at play is the peculiarly American notion of plastic as a symbol of our infinitely malleable selves, selves that can always be improved. If there is such a thing as a national trait, then the American national trait is self-improvement.

And there's something else too—a plastic ideology that used to be known as "rugged individualism" and then became one of "personal responsibility" has permeated our culture since the advent of capitalism. This ideology says that we are responsible for ourselves, and that we all have a chance to make it if we just work hard enough. In this case, the hard work of beauty becomes something we must all do, and if we don't, then we deserve our low pay, or lack of healthcare, or lonely, unmarried futures. It's an interesting ideology, and it grew up alongside capitalism to free the state from responsibility to the individual and make the individual see failure as a personal, not a structural, problem.

This is where my work is different from previous books on the meaning of plastic beauty. I am looking at culture and economy within the particular historical conditions of the United States. I agree with the feminist analysis that the explosion in cosmetic surgery is the result of a backlash against women, particularly white, middle-aged, middle-class women who claimed more power in the 1970s and 1980s. I also agree that plastic beauty is a way for modern citizens to actively express agency by acknowledging that beauty does have its advantages. But neither of these analyses is fully situated in the economy. Although Elliot places cosmetic surgery in the global economy, he misses the notion that plastic is ultimately a very American ideology, where people pull themselves up by their own bootstraps or back fat or whatever the future aphorism of the ideology of individualism will be.

And ultimately, it was not just American ideologies about self, but a self set loose in the wild frontiers of the global economy. This American ideology imagines the self as a free-floating agent, a sort of modern-day cowboy, who rides through the wide-open markets with no responsibility to anyone except the self, and no support from anyone or anything.[65] The fact that the ideologies of plastic and infinite opportunity are so out of touch with what most Americans were experiencing created a radical disjunction between beliefs and experiences. Even as we learned to work longer hours than people in other industrialized countries, and even as most of us were getting poorer, not richer, we clung to the belief in American plastic. But this disjuncture produced anxiety, and the anxiety had to express itself in a cultural form. That form was the insecurity of the body—especially the aging body.

CHAPTER 2

The State of Plastic

The American Dream

I'm sixty years old and I wanted a nice new face to go with my beautiful new life.

— BETTY FORD, on why she got a facelift

On a Friday morning in February of 2007, I, along with thousands of other Americans, shuffled through a security checkpoint to enter the Broward County Convention Center in Fort Lauderdale, Florida. The security check, set up along what used to be a road for vehicular traffic, baffled me. Why so much security for a convention center? Was it post-9/11 hysteria at its worst? Who would target the Broward County Convention Center? It's not like it's the Pentagon or some other symbol of American might.

But I think I understand now. On that day, my fellow convention goers and I *were* America. In other words, the Broward County Convention Center had managed to condense American identity and longing into a set of three events: an antique car show, a baby show, and a cosmetic surgery exposition. Upon entering the doors of the hulking cement monster of a building, we could gaze with awe and desire on a perfectly restored 1966 red Mustang, a brilliantly designed Swedish stroller that would fold into a neat package with a simple push of a button, and a plethora of silicone breast implants in a variety of shapes and sizes.

I searched the halls looking for differences between those who had come for the antique cars and those interested in diaper-disposal mechanisms. Could I tell them apart from those of us seeking information on the latest facelift? But it was dif-

ficult to distinguish one set of convention goers from another.
We all looked terribly ordinary—mostly white, mostly aging,
mostly appropriately gendered in tacky vacation wear. None of
us were especially well groomed; our midsections bulged. And
we all sought the same thing: perfection—perfect car, perfect
baby, perfect body.

It is the quest for perfection through consumption that is
the driving force of the American economy. Seventy percent
of our gross domestic product is based on consumption.[1] That
consumption is the result of many forces—TV, magazines, and
other cultural scripts—but it's also the result of very dramatic
changes in our economy and our politics. To borrow a phrase
from Bill Clinton's camp, we consume more and more cosmetic
surgery not just because of a culture that instructs us to do so,
but also because of "the economy, stupid!"

Consider a familiar example from the world of economics:
subprime mortgages. American culture teaches us to want to
be homeowners. Real families live in homes. Middle-class people want homes. Everybody wants a home. But it wasn't until
banks were allowed to create "financial products" like subprime
mortgages that targeted new groups of consumers that we began to see the dark side of the home-mortgage industry. As we
now know, subprime mortgages targeted first-time homeowners
who were disproportionately of color. Approximately 80 percent
of subprime mortgage holders were Black or Latino (versus 27
percent of the population).[2] Although 20 percent of subprime
mortgage holders would have qualified for regular mortgages,
they were pushed into debt vehicles with interesting new ways
of extracting wealth, like exploding interest rates. The result
was a huge amount of profit for the banks and a nightmare of
bankruptcy and foreclosure for Americans pursuing the dream.
In 2009 a quarter of all subprime loans were in foreclosure and
up to 5.8 million more homes were at risk of foreclosure.[3] Why
did they agree to such things? Were the people signing these

loans "greedy" or "stupid"? Probably not more so than any other Americans trying to get a better life. Probably no more than cosmetic surgery patients who take on medical credit. What they were was inexperienced and blatantly taken advantage of by the banks. Between 1994 and 2005, subprime loans went from a $35 billion to a $665 billion industry. This could happen because of a little thing the economists like to call "information asymmetry." In other words, the banks understood what all that fine print meant, but the homeowners did not.

But America's plastic economy also happened because the state stepped back from regulating how the banks make their profit. Letting banks charge any interest rate they wanted to began in the Reagan era. During that time, a body of laws was passed, including the 1980 Depository Institutions Deregulation and Monetary Control Act, which basically ended state regulation of banks. But the banks didn't really bet the bank on risky, high-interest forms of credit until the 1990s. By the 1990s, the financial situation of the majority of Americans was worse than it had been in 1980, and achieving the American dream seemed nearly impossible—taking on more debt at higher interest rates was the only way to make it. Within the logic of the time, you had to take risks to get ahead.[4]

Debt for cosmetic surgery is the subprime-mortgage crisis of the body. When it came to owning the perfect body, however, financial institutions targeted not urban homeowners but working- and middle-class white women. Medical credit companies and even the cosmetic surgeons who profited from them encouraged some Americans to take on large amounts of debt at extraordinarily high interest rates in pursuit of a better body as a path to a better life. But the economy and culture of both the subprime-mortgage industry and cosmetic surgery could never have happened without a political and ideological revolution in the United States that brought about the deregulation of credit and allowed medicine to become a for-profit enterprise. Letting more Americans assume greater debt—and simultaneously allowing medicine to sell itself—meant that plastic surgery was paid for with plastic money by Americans hoping that reshaping their bodies would reshape their lives. The revolution that set the stage for American plastic was both political and economic. The revolution was neoliberalism.

The Neoliberal Revolution

> *We are all Keynesians now.*
>
> — RICHARD NIXON

> *We are all neoliberals now.*
>
> — DAVID HARVEY, paraphrasing Richard Nixon

During the Great Depression, many politicians and economists became advocates of Keynesian economic policies. Keynesian economics, based on the ideas of John Maynard Keynes, stressed that the best way to keep capitalism thriving was with an active state—regulating the market and also spending money on creating a social safety net. All the New Deal programs that survived, including Social Security and Medicare, are products of Keynesian thinking. In the 1970s, as stagflation took hold and the great era of growth came to a close, Keynesian economics lost its grip on economists and politicians. A revolution, both political and economic, took place. This revolution created economic policies and an ideological climate that made the search for individual perfection not just possible, but necessary.

The economic revolution of the 1980s was based on a particular school of economic theory most often associated with Milton Friedman. Friedman, and the Chicago school of economics he propagated, believed that the New Deal and the social safety net it spun must be destroyed, since capitalism worked best when completely unfettered by government regulations.[5] This way of thinking is now called neoliberalism. In *A Brief*

History of Neoliberalism, cultural geographer David Harvey says the motivating ideology behind the policies of Ronald Reagan and Maggie Thatcher and the neoliberal revolution is the belief in the power of the individual and personal freedom. The individual has the "freedom of choice" to enter into a variety of contracts. The individual may enter into a contract with an employer, or the state, or even a cosmetic surgeon. In order for the individual to exercise this "freedom" effectively, there can be no state interference or regulation. In fact, states are reduced to facilitating markets by encouraging increased communication (the "information highway") and standardization (globalization). States must also actively suppress the demands of labor. By doing this, states create the conditions for markets to thrive and can thus justify privatizing that which was previously outside the market: schools, water, medicine. The motivating force behind neoliberalism is not greed, or at least not consciously, but the unshakable belief that "individual freedoms are guaranteed by freedom of the market and of trade."[6]

Neoconservative leaders let loose a whole set of policies that were meant to free the individual to operate in a market free from the state. These policies, Reaganomics or "trickle-down economics," were based on a simple idea: lower taxes for the rich and let the rich spend that money, thereby driving economic growth. The obvious corollary to this policy was to cut federal spending (on social, but not military, programs) in order to compensate for lost tax revenues. As the great neoliberal philosopher Reagan once put it, "More countries than ever before are following America's revolutionary economic message of free enterprise, low taxes, and open world trade. These days, whenever I see foreign leaders, they tell me about their plans for reducing taxes, and other economic reforms that they are using, copying what we have done here in our country."[7] While vacationing at his ranch in August of 1981, Reagan signed what might be the single most important piece of neoliberal economic legislation.

Reagan, looking suspiciously similar to one of the fictional Ewings—white cowboy hat, cowboy boots, spectacular wealth all
on display—signed the Economic Recovery Tax Act of 1981,
assuring us that we too could be as rich as the magical people
we watched on TV, if only we'd give more money to the rich.[8]
The result of this law and of trickle-down economics more
generally was not, however, wealth for most Americans. In fact,
when more money was given to the rich, they got richer, while
average Americans were left with fewer and fewer social services
and a labor movement that was consistently and purposefully opposed by the federal government. The result was that most Americans assumed more debt, and ultimately became much poorer.
Although the economy grew during most of this time, the wealth
was concentrated in the hands of fewer Americans. According to
the American Political Science Association's Task Force on Inequality and American Democracy, the U.S., Britain, and France
all managed to reduce inequality up until the 1970s, but the
United States changed dramatically so that by 1998, "the share of
income held by the very rich was two or three times higher in the
United States than in Britain and France."[9] A decade after Reagan
started giving tax breaks to the rich and deregulating industry,
the United States had the most unequal distribution of income of
any industrialized country in the world.[10]
Rising economic insecurity was met with a fiercely reinvigorated ideology of individual responsibility that led many Americans to seek "individual solutions" to their economic insecurity.
The economic revolution that Reagan espoused was based on the
idea that the individual, and the individual alone, is responsible
for his or her well-being. As Reagan also said, "Government
does not solve problems; it subsidizes them . . . The nine most
terrifying words in the English language are, 'I'm from the government and I'm here to help.'"[11] Within the ideology of neoliberalism, we were all supposed to believe that our problems were
ours and ours alone. One person's unemployment was a personal

issue. The unemployment of 15 million people was still a personal issue. One analysis of the rhetoric of neoliberalism found that "more and more, public issues became defined as personal troubles and problems of lifestyles."[12] In other words, the objective of state and society became to leave the individual alone to figure out how to get a better life. At the same time that the individual was "set free," for-profit industries, like medicine and banking, were also freed from state regulation, allowing them to more easily extract wealth from newly liberated individuals.

But this wasn't just a revolution from the top and for the top. The neoliberal belief that what's good for the rich is good for all of us found expression from the bottom and middle as well. As journalist Thomas Frank tells us in *What's the Matter with Kansas?* huge numbers of middle- and working-class Americans began to think that neoliberal economic policies were good for them (despite all evidence to the contrary). In a truly perverse move, the neoliberal dream of helping the rich through policies of trickle-down economics successfully sold itself to ordinary Americans as *anti-elitist*. The Rush Limbaughs and Glenn Becks as well as the George Bushes and Ronald Reagans of the world were seen as "regular Joes" and for the "common guy."[13] The fact that the economic policies unleashed from the top had popular support from below means that the American body—the body politic and the literal body—became hostage to this new order. By making most people less secure economically, by deregulating medicine, and by allowing the banking industry to create new forms of credit, neoliberalism ended up written on the bodies of ordinary Americans as plastic surgery.

Shopping for the American Dream

The marriage of pro-business economic policies with the popular acceptance of the ideological claims of neoliberalism meant that, rather than looking to things like regulating the cost of healthcare or mandating livable wages for workers, we Americans were drawn to perfecting ourselves and our surroundings. We decided that the best response to economic insecurity was to go shopping. Americans believed that the best way to guarantee our future security was not through collective action, but the individual projects of creating the perfect home, the perfect kitchen, the perfect child, or the perfect body.

Of course, as an economic strategy, shopping for a better life might have been a rational response at first. But shopping became an inefficient response to financial instability once everyone tried to buy the American dream. As economist Robert H. Frank puts it,

> to the extent that wearing the right suit, driving the right car, wearing the right watch, or living in the right neighborhood may help someone land the right job . . . these expenditures are more like investments than true consumption. But from the collective vantage point, they are extremely inefficient investments, for when we all spend more their return falls to zero.[14]

Or, to put it another way, if more and more of us are buying fake breasts and wrinkle-free faces, then investing in such things will no longer increase our competitive edge.

But we were trapped. We knew we were getting poorer. The future was not bright. But we also understood it was our fault. Rich people deserve their wealth. If you're not rich, or even financially secure, it's your own fault. If only we were more like them. If only we had better stuff and better bodies. We were drawn to places like the Broward County Convention Center like moths to a flame. In the space of the convention hall, we could imagine a better future if only we could buy that car, that stroller, or those breast implants. Success could only happen through individual action. And what could be more individual, more engaged in the nearly universal belief that we are all responsible for ourselves, than reshaping our bodies? The rugged individual of neoliberalism melted into the standardized body of cosmetic surgery. Newly plastic Americans operated within a strangely warped neoliberal belief that a body more standardized and less individual would lead to a better job, a better husband, and a better life.

Plastic Medicine

Feel good. Get the breasts you've always dreamed about.
—From a billboard ad for breast-enhancement surgery

Not only did the politics of America change as the neoliberal revolution took hold, but the policies changed as well, as the state stepped back from any responsibility for the market's excesses. Two events in the early years of the Reagan administration changed plastic surgery forever: allowing medical professionals to advertise their services, and allowing banks to extend credit to more and more people by allowing them to charge whatever interest rate the market could bear.

In 1982 the Supreme Court upheld an earlier Federal Trade Commission (FTC) ruling that doctors should be allowed to advertise.[15] Although there were medical advertisements before this, American Medical Association (AMA)–approved physicians were not allowed to advertise. This was because the AMA aimed to professionalize medicine by distinguishing "real" doctors from "quacks," and therefore did not allow any of its members to "solicit patients." The FTC argued, using the logic of neoliberalism, that medicine, too, would benefit from the magic of the market because advertising would give patients the information they needed to make informed decisions about their medical care. The Supreme Court agreed.[16] After 1982, all physicians, but especially cosmetic surgeons, advertised. Cosmetic surgery had always been voluntary, and this made "patients" far more like "customers." If a plastic surgeon couldn't give you the best service at the best price, you could just go elsewhere. But advertising made plastic surgery more visible to potential consumers and even more visibly a business. Advertising changed the way we think of plastic surgery, from a medical relationship between a surgeon and a patient, to a commercial relationship between a consumer and a service provider. Boob jobs are advertised on billboards; at least for now, cancer treatments are not.

Advertising is the art of promising magical transformation through a particular form of consumption. Cosmetic surgeons have their own sort of magic: a little sleight of hand known as "before and after." As anyone who has even glanced at the before and after photos knows, plastic surgery advertisements suck the viewer in with the promise of any fairytale: a not terribly attractive woman (sometimes a man) is turned into a younger, thinner, more beautiful self with the wave of a wand/scalpel. The American Society of Plastic Surgeons (ASPS) keeps a large collection of before and after photos on its Web site,[17] as do all the medical credit companies, so anyone considering cosmetic surgery has probably looked at them. But we have all been bombarded with these images in the newspapers we read and on the computer social-networking sites we use. In advertising for cosmetic surgery, sagging breasts are transformed into perky ones, flat buttocks are made bodacious, wrinkles are erased, tummies tucked, the old made young, and the fat, thin.

With the technological wonders of computer imaging, before and after photographs can now be produced without any actual surgery. Now surgeons and potential consumers of cosmetic surgery can submit a photograph to places like Angels Lab and get a "realistic" image back of a postsurgical face or body part. According to the Angels Lab Web site, such computer imaging "can help you determine if a cosmetic procedure is right for you."[18] Some surgeons have this sort of equipment right in their offices. "This is what your nose/breasts/stomach would look like if you just sign on the dotted line" makes plastic surgeons resemble the fairy godmothers of commercialized medicine. With a wave of their magic scalpels, they can turn ugly ducklings into swans. Unlike fairy godmothers, however, the surgeons and the banks will make a nice profit off the transformation.

Despite the entrepreneurial spirit of many doctors, quite a few plastic surgeons are troubled by these before and after photos and the sleight of hand they represent. Advertisements elevate patient expectations that "miracles are possible," though the operating room tends to produce more ordinary results. Two Dallas, Texas, cosmetic surgeons actually educate their patients about why they should not believe in before and after photographs. "Before and After Pictures: Seeing is Believing . . . or is it? Publicly displayed before and after pictures (ads, marketing seminars or internet) may help you make the decision to have cosmetic surgery but they may not be the best way to select a surgeon."[19]

Many of the surgeons I interviewed were uneasy about the marriage of advertising and medicine in their industry. Several surgeons pointed out that when people are paying for a procedure over time, they're more likely to be dissatisfied with the results. This was only exacerbated by the "unrealistic expectations" people get from advertising. One surgeon said, "Women come in and want huge breasts. They want Double Ds that are perky, that stand straight up." These surgeons are engaged in a different form of salesmanship, of course. They're offering "realistic" results and are therefore not "charlatans." But their concern that advertising is not necessarily a good thing for their industry is also real.

Whether cosmetic surgeons like advertising, it exists, and more or less without any regulation of its truthfulness. And the surgeons are not organizing to regulate it. "Caveat emptor" was the attitude of many surgeons I interviewed. They most certainly did not want the federal government to step in. As a San Francisco–based surgeon I spoke to remarked, "Consumers have to be somewhat savvy. They've got to do their research." This sort of claim is, of course, at the center of neoliberal America. The doctor's only responsibility is to make a profit. The patient is a consumer, and as a consumer, buyer beware. Just because the doctor might understand the credit system better than the eighteen-year-old minimum-wage worker who comes into the office doesn't mean the doctor has a responsibility to tell the patient not to use it. It's their "choice," after all.

The ability of surgeons to aggressively market their magic through advertising is one of the major reasons we are buying more and more plastic surgery. Some plastic surgeons may not like advertising, but *all* of them are benefiting from it. According to the American Society of Plastic Surgeons, advertising is one of the major reasons that by 2015, about 17 percent of the U.S. population will get some sort of cosmetic work done.[20] But how will we pay for it?

Plastic Money

Credit, like prescription drugs or automobiles or meat, is one of those high-value, high-risk products that need to be regulated.
— JOSE GARCIA, JAMES LARDNER, and CINDY ZELDIN

I have no idea where my patients get the money to pay me. I don't know and I don't care.
— PLASTIC SURGEON to author, May 2008

We pay for our new, plastic selves with plastic money, of course. Customers pay with traditional credit cards, but they also pay by way of medical credit companies that specialize in financing elective surgeries. Here's a typical one from a Web site called Make Me Heal:

> You don't have to put off your plans for a plastic surgery or a non-surgical cosmetic treatment. Designed specifically for plastic surgery patients, our Finance Me Program will enable you to pay for any type of cosmetic procedure with low, easy, and convenient monthly payments at interest rates that are comparable to or lower than most major credit cards . . . No

down payment is required and we can finance loans as low as
$1,000 and up to $25,000 . . . We specialize in providing financing for patients with all types of credit profiles.[21]

You don't need to put off your surgery, but you also won't be
able to put off the high-interest monthly payments that will
come with it.

A 2005 poll conducted by the American Society of Plastic
Surgeons found that 30 percent of plastic surgery patients earned
less than $30,000 a year, while another 41 percent earned be-
tween $31,000 and $60,000.[22] One surgeon, from a very blue-
collar town in California, where the unemployment rate is about
twice the national average, framed it like this: "There's a fallacy
in the public. They think it's all rich people who do aesthetic
procedures. But my patients have jobs, regular jobs and know
the value of money. They price shop. They're teachers and real
estate agents and bankers, but they're also people in entry-level
jobs working in the mall."

Another surgeon, this one from New York State, told me:
"My patients are not what you'd expect demographically. I don't
practice in Miami or Dallas. A lot of my patients work in bars.
But if you're a woman who has a few kids and you've taken care
of yourself, but lost a lot of volume in your breasts, we can fix it
. . . And if you lost half your money in the bank, is it better to
invest in the bank or yourself?"

As these quotes illustrate, plastic surgery, once only for the
wealthiest Americans, is now available to the rest of us not because we are getting richer, but because we have more and more
opportunities to take on debt.

Medical credit for plastic surgery is big business for the
banks, which are financing not just cosmetic surgery,[23] but also
cosmetic dentistry and veterinary bills. Since the deregulation
of the industry, banks no longer rely on actual money or equity
to make their profit. Instead, the bulk of their money is made
from interest rates and fees. This "financialization" of the bank-

ing industry, where it's no longer about equity but rather financial products, created unprecedented profits for banks. Between 1990 and 2005, bank profits increased 400 percent.[24] Even after the economic collapse of 2007, banks have managed to stay profitable by charging higher interest rates and fees.[25]

The banking industry is not just making a lot of money off credit; they actually make more money off poor people than rich people. Under the guiding principles of Chicago school economics, credit was opened up to all sorts of people who previously did not have access to it: students and retirees, then the working poor, and by the 1990s, even the recently bankrupt. But since these people were "risky," credit rates had to adjust accordingly. Miss a payment or have a bad credit history and your interest rate balloons up to nearly 30 percent. That means that if you're poor, you might end up paying double for your $8,000 boob job over the course of five years of paying it off. That's not surprising. That's how credit, in unregulated markets, works. In the unregulated market, the credit industry is able to squeeze profit from some of the poorest members of society like blood from a turnip. The Federal Reserve estimated that in 2004 a working-class family (household income less than $30,000 a year) paid 56.1 percent more on an auto loan than a wealthy family (household earning more than $90,000) did.[26] In other words, boobs, like cars and home mortgages, cost more for the poor than the rich. And if you somehow managed to pay this exorbitant interest rate by making yourself sick working all the time, no worries: your friends in medical credit are increasingly willing to pay for lifesaving medical treatment, like insulin and hospital stays, for the 47 million uninsured Americans and the 16 million underinsured Americans. The result is a lot of profit for credit companies charging the highest interest rates that the market will bear to "help" poor and working-class Americans get medical care so that they can live, and facelifts so that they can dream.[27]

In the cosmetic surgery medical-credit world, the most powerful medical credit company is General Electric's CareCredit,
which in 2007 was worth about $5 billion and had risen 40
percent from the year before.[28] CareCredit's Web site describes
the company's services this way:

> Maybe you'd like a brighter smile or better vision. Maybe
> you want to freshen your look. Or maybe your family pet
> needs a surgery you didn't plan for . . . CareCredit, a GE
> Money Company, gives you convenient payment options so
> you can get the procedure you want, when you want it . . .
> CareCredit gives you the freedom to get your procedure
> whenever you're ready . . . you can say goodbye to the wait-
> ing time and reward yourself sooner.[29]

The CareCredit Web site lists the annual interest rate at
13.90 percent, which means that if you took out a sixty-month
loan to pay for your $8,000 breast implants, you would end up
paying over $11,000. What the Web site doesn't make clear is
that if you miss a payment, the interest rate could more than
double. The Web site also doesn't explain that the doctors who
use CareCredit's services are also charged, on top of what the
patient is charged. The cosmetic surgeon then passes the cost of
doing business with medical credit companies onto the patient
in the form of higher fees.

A Beverly Hills cosmetic surgeon, a man in his late sixties
who tells me he has performed thirty-two thousand nose jobs,
had this to say about the practice:

> Medical credit is a good example of how the rich have gotten
> richer because of the deregulation of banking. And the poor
> poorer . . .
>   Using medical credit is stupid for surgeons and patients.
> These companies are often charging us surgeons 5 percent on

top of what they've already charged the patient. So they get breast implants for $8,000 and they end up paying $12,500? It's so stupid. The banks and other middlemen are making the money and these big corporations that back them, like GE . . . I get a check from GE! But sometimes they'll say they can't pay me because the patient isn't paying them. Really? A huge corporation like GE can't pay me? . . .

But these guys [bankers] get all the breaks. Look what we're doing now. We're bailing out the bankers when they're the ones who screwed everything up. No one bails me out if I screw up.

Plastic surgeons are charging more for their procedures in order to pay for the medical credit service so that megacorporations like GE can extract profit twice from patients who can ill afford it the first time. Even as a successful Beverly Hills surgeon profits from the system of medical credit, he understands that it is not to his patients' benefit.

General Electric is not alone in getting into the more marginal practices of lending. Money for people who don't have money is big business these days. Bank of America has about $110 million in the quickly expanding "payday loan" business, a system whereby financially strapped Americans can get cash in exchange for future paychecks at what is an annual interest rate of 390 percent.[30] In comparison, CareCredit's rate of up to 28.5 percent looks like a far better investment. One of the ways GE and other corporations have stayed profitable during the economic downturn is to refuse to finance some populations. A plastic surgeon from Las Vegas, a white man in his fifties who describes his patients as nearly all women and nearly all working in the "adult entertainment or tourism" industry, complained that CareCredit stopped financing his patients in 2008 as credit dried up for many Americans.

Some may see this as a luxury, but for these women it's less luxury and more necessity, not just fun, but an investment. These women are jockeying for their jobs . . . Listen, you're a professor. You know that people go to college to get a better job, not a beautiful education. And getting surgery is about getting a better job. Or keeping a job.

Another major player in the medical credit industry, Capital One, had to get out of the medical credit business entirely to maintain its profit margin of $453 million in 2008 (down from $750 million the year before). The number one reason for Capital One's declining profits was consumers not being able to pay off their loans. The percentage of loans in default nearly doubled to 6.26 percent during the same time.[31] Apparently Capital One, which tended to charge lower interest rates to patients and did not double charge by tacking a fee onto the surgeon as well, just wasn't extracting enough wealth from poor and working-class Americans to make medical credit worth its while. But there are a variety of medical credit companies still willing to provide plastic money for plastic surgery. That's good news for the majority of patients I spoke with, since most of them were definitely considering financing their surgeries.

One woman who was fifty-six and considering a tummy tuck because she'd had a C-section years ago and didn't like the way her stomach looked, weighed the costs of surgery: "Sure I'm concerned about the risks, but I'm more concerned about the money. Some of my friends have had it done for like $8,000 and others for $12,000 . . . I'm considering financing half of it. I mean, it would be one of the stupider things, since it's not like it's medically necessary."

The husband of a cosmetic surgery patient told me he had spent $20,000 on his wife's procedures. Not that he thought she needed them, especially at her age (seventy). "It's way too much money and it's money poorly spent. There are all these old people in trailers and crappy apartments who haven't planned for their retirement and they think they have the money to spend on this?" I asked why he agreed to the expense. "To make my wife happy. She's in the fashion industry. Has been for forty years. And it's all about first impressions in that business."

Another woman, thirty-nine, who wanted a body lift told me she'd have to finance it because she's single, self-employed, and has two kids. When I asked her if she worried about the risks, health or financial, associated with the procedure, she said, "Whatever it takes to look good is worth it. . . . I don't really think about it. At least I'm taking a chance on something, on making my life better, to look good."

In other words, risks are necessary to succeed in the United States. If you're not successful, then you haven't taken the right risks. It has nothing to do with an unfair system. Anyone can make it if they just work harder, go under the knife, and take out more debt.

American Plastic

It's important to note just how American the idea is that it's "worth it" to take out a huge amount of debt for better boobs. Only in the land of endless optimism and self-improvement can large numbers of people believe that the way out of poverty and dead-end jobs is to take on high-interest loans to reshape the body. Based on the responses of plastic surgeons from over twenty countries and five continents, few other countries have a similar credit industry devoted to the purchase of aesthetic procedures. Although many countries have credit card systems similar to the United States', most do not have interest rates as high as the American average of 18.9 percent plus fees.[32] The only countries that I found that had similar systems of high-interest medical credit were Mexico and Australia. As one surgeon from Mexico City told me, "We have a lot of people from the U.S. and Canada who come to Mexico for surgeries. Most of my patients are from the North. And they use their own medical credit, but we have the same credit system. There's no difference. So when the U.S. credit market collapsed, it hurt us too." However, with the exception of these countries, no other surgeons described anything like the surgery-specific credit industries that we have in the United States. And no doctors told me that they work directly with the medical credit companies, a common practice among U.S. plastic surgeons.

A Toronto surgeon, whose practice is 100 percent aesthetic and therefore not covered by Canada's government healthcare system, told me that the vast majority of his patients are not wealthy. They're teachers, secretaries, or staff at one of the universities, and many often take a line of credit from their banks. The interest rates are not nearly as high as those found in the United States, however, and patients in Toronto must have some equity to pay with credit. "Canada is different from the U.S.," he said. "You need to put twenty-five percent down to get a mortgage. People are not living on the edge in the same way in Canada as in the U.S."

A surgeon from Seoul, South Korea, had a similar observation: "In my country the situation is different. People pay with cash or credit card, but the credit card interest rates are 2.5 to 3 percent. And we have none of these medical credit companies you have here." A surgeon from Argentina described his practice as an all-cash business: "We have no credit in Argentina. Everyone has to pay cash. There's no credit available to anyone. I need to pay with cash. If I want to buy some equipment here I have to arrange it with my bank, arrange for cash."

A Swiss plastic surgeon, practicing at the absolute center of the world banking industry, laughed when I asked him if there were similar high-interest medical credit companies in Switzerland. "There is no credit for this in Switzerland. The government regulates such things. We surgeons have to get the money up front because it's not covered by insurance. Sometimes insurance will pay for a breast reduction, but for our patients breast implants are the most popular procedure."

Many of the American plastic surgeons wanted a different system, but the system they imagined was one of savvier consumers and more ethical colleagues. A lot of them expressed concern that their profession had become a completely unregulated market. One surgeon said that using medical credit often led to more dissatisfaction, since "every time [plastic surgery patients] write a check, especially if there were any complications, they think 'I can't believe I'm still paying for this.'"

Another surgeon commented:

Debt-free living, it's not possible in this country. I can't do it. I don't know anyone who can. I only have one friend from college who is debt free. But to be what I am, to have built up my business, I had to take on debt . . .

But I do not like it when I see these high school girls coming in for breast implants. And they live in a trailer park. And their parents finance them for them. So they pay $6,600 instead of the $3,300 it was supposed to cost.

Surgeons often blamed the commercialization of cosmetic surgery on the new generation of surgeons: "These kids are coming out of Harvard and doing these three-stitch facelifts! They know damn well it won't last but all they care about is building up their business. It's like these new McMansions you see being built everywhere. It's the same people living in them."

One surgeon lamented the fact that his field was so commodified:

What have we come to as a culture that patients are willing to do this no matter what? This is what America's about. It's all about me. . . . We're not willing to sacrifice. We've borrowed and borrowed. Look, don't take a mortgage you can't afford just assuming the value of your home will go up forever. . . . This country has fallen off the deep end.

But I don't look at cosmetic surgery as bad though, because we can safely enhance people, making them look better, and there's nothing wrong with that . . . the government should let me say, I'll do your operation for a minimal amount plus fifty hours of community service [and] then I'd get a tax benefit.

Unlike this last respondent, most American plastic surgeons, like their patients, saw the solutions as outside state regulation and in individual responses. Because surgeons, patients, and finance companies alike all rely on the neoliberal rhetoric of "individual choice," no one can imagine a time when individuals cannot "choose" to take on high levels of debt to reshape their bodies. For the surgeons and the lending companies, such a time would result in far fewer customers and far less profit for them.

And so the American dream of ever-expanding opportunity is alive and well. Can't afford a boob job? Take out this loan and don't worry, because things will only get better. You can pay it off in the future, when your boob job pays off with a better job or a better husband. And who was seduced by this promise of a better future through plastic consumption? We all were, in one form or another, because we all were seduced by the promise of perfection. As I explore in the next chapter, Americans were drawn to different sorts of consumption: some of us wanted boobs, others wanted cars. But for nearly everyone, the American dream as imagined within neoliberalism was reduced to different forms of plastic consumption.

CHAPTER 3

Plastic People and Their Doctors

This is probably obvious, since I'm writing a book on plastic surgery, but I am ridiculously vain. So vain, in fact, that I don't want to be confused with "those people"—the ones who are plastic. That's why when I arrived at my first cosmetic surgery conference, I was extremely anxious to get my media badge. The little plastic badge with my name and the word PRESS underneath it was like a magical talisman that would protect me from plastic infection. Sadly, there would be no magic bullet against plastic that first morning. In my field notes I wrote: *Arrrggghhh!!!! Press office closed. Now I have to walk around with everyone thinking I'm here because I want plastic surgery. Maybe they'll think I'm a plastic surgeon. Is that better?* There I was, naked, with no protection from becoming a plastic person myself.

I walked resolutely into the conference hall, notebook in hand, hoping it would inoculate me against plastic. I took a deep breath and began to ask a plastic surgeon a few questions. The surgeon was a very attractive white man in his thirties. He looked slightly overdressed, his expensive suit out of place in a somewhat tasteless exhibition booth for Botox. His office manager, a voluptuous Latina in a tight skirt, high heels, and a white satin blouse unbuttoned just enough to reveal two perfect implants, stood next to him. I introduced myself as a sociologist and writer; in other words, as a person who was most certainly not plastic. Five minutes into the interview, the doctor poked at the bags under my eyes.

"You should really get some Botox now or you're going to need a major facelift in ten years."

"Hmm," I responded, hoping to sound as if I didn't care about such superficial things as bags under my eyes. "Can I ask you some more questions?" I continued, trying to reassert my professional authority as "the interviewer," not "the patient."

"OK, but are you really not going to do anything about those nasolabial folds?" he prodded. "You don't want to end up looking like a marionette."

At this point, I was forty-one-years old. Since turning forty I had been trying to maintain an internal mantra of "It's OK to be an aging woman." The mantra came to a screeching halt.

"Marionette? Like Punch and Judy?" I gasped. The truth that my aging face was slowly morphing into Judy's hit me like a punch to the gut, making it difficult to breathe.

"I don't know who that is," the young doctor glibly replied, my cultural reference to a long-ago show clearly marking me as far more aged than he.

Virginia Blum, who experienced similar disruptions to her professional status when she tried to interview plastic surgeons, believes that plastic surgeons cannot stop themselves from offering their professional opinions, since "they see us all with an aesthetic gaze that is additionally a transformative gaze—what they can do for the defective face and body."[1] I knew from that point on that I, too, could not help myself. No professional status as "press" or "professor" could protect me from the hypnotic spell of being told what was wrong with my body and what could be done to fix it.

Between February 2007 and May 2009 I attended four conferences of cosmetic surgeons and their patients: an exposition for potential consumers of cosmetic surgery in February of 2007 in Fort Myers, Florida; a meeting of the American Society for Aesthetic Plastic Surgery (ASAPS) in May of 2007 in New York City and again in May of 2009 in Las Vegas; and a congress of the International Confederation for Plastic, Reconstructive, and Aesthetic Surgery (IPRAS) in June of 2007 in Berlin. In all, I interviewed sixty-nine cosmetic surgeons. Of these, four-teen were women. Thirty-four of the surgeons were from North America (thirty-two from the United States, one from Canada, and one from Mexico). The rest were from the European Union (ten), Eastern Europe or the former Soviet Union (six), Asia (four), South America (six), the Middle East (five), and Austra-lia/New Zealand (four). Of the thirty-four North American doc-tors I interviewed, almost all were men (twenty-nine) and white (twenty-eight).

I conducted both participant observation and formal inter-views at the cosmetic surgery exposition. Through four days of participant observation, I informally spoke with 137 people in-terested in getting cosmetic surgery. Often these people were in groups of two to four friends or family members. I also con-ducted formal interviews that ranged from twenty-five minutes to an hour with twenty-eight patients or potential patients of cosmetic surgery. Of these, most were women (twenty-four) and most were white (one Asian American woman and three Latinas). The patients I interviewed were between twenty and eighty years old, but most were between thirty-five and fifty.

Although hardly a perfect representation of who *gets* cos-metic surgery and who *performs* cosmetic surgery, the gender and racial makeup of patients is not that different from the gen-eral patterns we saw in the previous chapter. About 86 percent of the patients I interviewed were female and 86 percent were white. The makeup of the surgeons is also fairly representative. Although women make up half of all medical students, only about 20 percent of them will do their residency in surgery.[2] Among cosmetic surgeons, an even higher percentage are men.[3] Furthermore, most surgeons in the United States are white (74 percent), versus about 11 percent Asian American, 3 percent African American, and 3.6 percent Latino.[4]

I also interviewed eleven vendors working in the field of cosmetic beauty products (six women and five men). In addition, I spoke with two journalists who regularly cover cosmetic surgery in their reporting to discuss their understanding of the cosmetic surgery industry. I also interviewed one man who runs a medical-tourism Web site for Americans who want to travel to other countries for cheaper cosmetic surgery. In addition to the interviews and participant observation, I attended over twenty informational sessions by producers of cosmetic products and/or scientific presentations by surgeons about cosmetic procedures.

So it is that in the past few years I have spent a lot of time with plastic people and their doctors. I no longer worry about making sure everyone knows I am "press." I suppose like any good anthropologist living among the colorful inhabitants of a foreign land, I have "gone native" and become plastic. Or perhaps I realized that there was never any real difference between "them" and me in the first place. I had been living in the land of plastic all along.

Plastic People

Not only did I imagine myself as different from plastic surgery patients, I also thought that plastic surgery patients were different from me. I thought they'd be so much more attractive than I am, so much more engaged in the task of "looking good," that I would look completely out of place among them. Nothing could be further from the truth. Plastic surgery patients look extraordinarily ordinary. They wear bad clothes, get bad haircuts, their dye jobs often reveal gray hairs, and they have excess weight in all sorts of places. In short, plastic people look like average Americans, because average Americans are plastic. Furthermore, they come to want plastic surgery for the exact same reasons any of us invest in anything: because they think it will make their lives better and more secure than they are now.

Plastic surgery patients felt their insecurity as both financial and emotional. Insecurity in the job market, insecurity in the romance market, and consumption of cultural texts that implant the idea that plastic surgery will make things better, drive average Americans to plastic beauty. And the desire for plastic surgery drives Americans to the plastic money to pay for it. As the potential patients entered the exposition, they were greeted by a variety of products for a "new and improved" version of themselves. Salespeople and surgeons offered attendees free advice on what they needed to do to look and feel better. They enticed them with free chocolate, free shopping bags, free T-shirts, even free videos of the sort of lipo they do, or a "new" sort of facelift.

One plastic surgeon, Alan Lefkin, performed "LIVE Botox Demonstrations," choosing people from the audience to demonstrate how "painless" and "effective" Botox is. In addition to the products, there were "educational" presentations on the sorts of procedures available, as well as what's wrong with modern (female, aging) bodies. For instance, audience members could attend a presentation on "breast ptosis," that is, the natural and inevitable sag of middle-aged breasts that has now been made into a medical condition and marked as a "problem" that can only be fixed by implants and lifts. Other doctors showed aging female faces with the problems of "wrinkles" or "sagging eyelids" or visibly sun-damaged skin.

Middle-aged mothers came in with their twenty-year-old daughters looking for facelift/boob job double dates. Young families with toddlers in tow fingered the latest breast implants as they weighed their cost against the plumbing fixtures they also wanted to buy. Girlfriends read through Botox and Juvéderm pamphlets, discussing whether they should invest in temporary measures or just do a facelift in a few years. Retirees, often veterans of plastic, talked about the boob job they did twenty years ago, or getting yet another facelift, or finally having the time and money to invest more in themselves. The shopping around was no different from buying a new pair of shoes. It was a way of bonding through a common consumption pattern—

the ultimate American socialization ritual. These slightly bulky, slightly aged Americans, the women in pastel-colored velour jogging suits, the men in Hawaiian shirts, spoke of their post-surgical futures as safer and happier than their insecure present.

Insecure Economy

Almost all of the patients I interviewed described plastic surgery as a response to economic insecurity. As we saw in the previous chapter, most economic indicators point to the downward mobility of the vast majority of Americans over the past twenty-five years. Indeed, as income for the top 1 percent of Americans has grown exponentially, the bottom 80 percent have seen a decrease in real wages as well as a decrease in the possibility of upward economic mobility. Not surprisingly, women of all races (and nonwhite men) were the most likely to experience decreasing wages and opportunities.[5]

Freda, a fifty-something white woman who is married, has two grown children, and owns her own business, told me that even as a self-employed person, she feels the need to look younger to get more customers: "More and more women are in the workplace, and now we [women] have to compete to look younger and younger and more fit. So I figured why not check [plastic surgery] out."

Rita, a white woman in her fifties who works in the hospitality industry, said she considered cosmetic surgery an "investment in my career." In the workplace today, she explained: "It's about how you look, not what you do. I do believe that nine times out of ten, women with the hot bodies get the best jobs, go further."

Adam, a young white man in his thirties, argued that Americans are getting poorer all the time, but because of credit and celebrity, we turn to plastic beauty as the answer.

There's a class of the superwealthy that's out there that we never used to know about, but now we see them everyday on

TV . . . People are living in mansions yet living paycheck by paycheck. I think there's some hopelessness out there. There are people who've run up a lot of debt because they know they're going to have to declare bankruptcy and they think why not get plastic surgery. But this is happening because people are hopeless. Thirty years ago people felt they could build a better life. It's getting harder and harder to cross the class divide.

People getting plastic surgery in hopes of securing a better economic future are not delusional. They understand that looks really do matter. Whether or not investing in cosmetic procedures will pay off in direct financial benefits is a different question, however. It depends on whether the surgery is paid for with a high-interest loan or in cash. It depends on what opportunity costs were lost by spending income on surgery rather than other paths to success, like education. But most importantly, it depends on the systems in which a person operates. Within American culture, a person's race, socioeconomic status, and geographic location have far more to do with "getting ahead" than the size and perkiness of one's breasts.

Ultimately, seeking an individual solution to a set of structural constraints can only go so far. As C. Wright Mills explained it in *The Sociological Imagination,* "people do not usually define the troubles they endure in terms of historical change and institutional contradiction," and yet our lives are always structured by these larger forces. For Mills, a single unemployed person is an individual problem, but 15 million unemployed people is a social issue.[6] A single set of sagging, aging breasts is an individual problem; a nation of them is a social issue. "If I just had better boobs, then I wouldn't be at the bottom of my pay scale" may seem like the thinking of a rational person, Homo economicus. But the truth is, plastic boobs or not, a structure of unfair pay and unfair opportunity is not going to disappear because of an individual's consumption patterns and body work. Still, a rational actor like Homo economicus might argue that even if the plastic surgery doesn't pay off financially, it will surely lead to a more satisfying romantic life, considering the premium placed on "looks."

Insecurity in the Romance Market

On Valentine's Day, a local spa advertised a special discount on Botox injections. The advertisement displayed a woman lying down with her eyes closed. A hand holding a syringe hovers over her face. Above her floats a cupid with a quiverful of arrows, waiting to shoot her full of true love, or facial paralysis, or perhaps both. The message is clear: love will come to those whose faces are smooth and wrinkle-free. Americans getting plastic surgery are not just feeling insecurity in the job market; they are also insecure in the romance market, a set of relationships that are often financial in nature, but also include a desire for emotional fulfillment outside of familial and friendship networks.

Romance is the most pervasive ideology of American culture. Americans spend an average of $26,327 on their weddings, an increase of 73 percent in the past fifteen years, making weddings, like plastic surgery in the United States, "recession proof."[7] American films and music are filled with the story of "true love" and happy endings. Even American politicians must construct a believable narrative of romance with their spouse, a romance that can survive dalliances with interns and escort services.[8] But the perfect romance, like the perfect body, is a promise eternally delayed. About half of all marriages will end in divorce; there are more single Americans than married ones, and unmarried American women are the fastest-growing segment of the population.[9] Faced with the disconnect between the ideology of romance and the reality of our lives, many Americans are turning to plastic surgery as a path to true love.

Research by Deborah Davis and Michael L. Vernon has

shown that people with a high level of anxiety over whether or not they're in a relationship are more likely to get cosmetic surgery. These people with high levels of "attachment anxiety" will do body work in an effort to either stay in an existing relationship or find a partner.[10] It is this hope that plastic surgery clients express over and over again when they say, "If I were married, I wouldn't need to get this done." Toni, a fifty-five-year-old white woman who works as an aesthetician, had a tummy tuck and a breast augmentation in her thirties. Two years ago, she had her first facelift. Now she's considering a breast reconstruction to counter the inevitable downward pull of gravity. "It's very, very hard as you get older," she explains. "Models and all this crap you see in the magazines. By the time you're fifty, you might as well be dead. If I was married, then nah, I wouldn't be doing this. If my husband loved me the way I was, but that's not reality, is it?"

Beth and her friend Linda, both mid-thirties white woman in the banking industry, spoke about plastic surgery as a necessary fix for a failed romance:

BETH: I'm not saying I wouldn't get certain things. I've gained weight, but I'm not ready for lipo, but maybe if I were older, in my forties . . . and men are continuously attracted to younger women and younger women are really so stupid, they'll go out with these guys.

LINDA: Inner beauty is not really focused on anymore. You're judged on how you look.

BETH: It was the same a hundred years ago, then it was corsets and bustles and now it's a boob job and lipo . . . If you're a 45-year-old woman and your husband has left you for a younger woman, well you've gotta find another man. The fact is a lot of women want a man who has money. They're successful men in business and they want some arm candy. Let me tell you, there are a lot of single women who might have stayed in their marriages if their husbands hadn't left them [for a younger woman]. My husband happens to be six years younger than me. I have friends whose husbands have left them for younger women . . . We have a friend [whose husband left her] and three years later she is still despondent. Not dating. Not concerned about how she looks, and you gotta be . . . or you'll be alone.

Adam echoed the understanding of plastic surgery as a fix for failed romance. "If I were single, maybe I'd do something. Look at my hair! I'm losing it. But I'm married, I'm confident enough."

Like job insecurity, romantic insecurity might be helped at an individual level by consuming cosmetic surgery. The individual, however, will not solve the larger contradictions of marriage, divorce, and individual desire through a single marriage, since that marriage, like all marriages, will be subject to a variety of societal pressures and limitations that make "happily ever after" a fairy tale.

When I asked why Americans are increasingly driven to cosmetic surgery, the answers were surprisingly similar: fear of aging and a culture that normalizes such measures, not to mention a mass media that makes us want to be young forever and tells us that the path to eternal youth is plastic surgery. In other words, the patients understood exactly why they were there, even if such self-awareness did nothing to interrupt the desire to go under the knife.

Aging and Youth-Obsessed Boomers

It's the aging baby boomers.

The baby boomers, we said we'd never get old and now we are getting old, so this is what we do.

It's definitely the baby boomers.

The baby boomers are not *growing old gracefully.*
> —Answers to the question, Why has there
> been such an increase in cosmetic surgery?

Plastic surgery patients, many of whom are part of the baby boom generation, saw the youth culture that their generation pioneered coupled with the aging bodies of late middle age as the real cause of the increase in cosmetic surgery. According to the National Institutes of Health, the number of Americans over sixty-five will double in the next two decades. By 2030, 20 percent of all Americans will be sixty-five or older. The age group eighty-five and older is now one of the fastest-growing segments of the U.S. population. Not only are a growing number of us going to be old, but we're also going to be healthier and wealthier than previous generations of old folks. Fewer older Americans are disabled by disease, and only about 10 percent of older Americans live in poverty, compared to more than a third in 1959.[11]

For many of the cosmetic surgery patients I interviewed, the cosmetic surgery industry is an excellent solution to the crisis caused by an aging yet still youth-obsessed generation. A white man who works in law enforcement pointed out that "people aren't just living longer, they're feeling younger than they used to. I'm fifty now and it used to be fifty was sitting on a porch in your rocking chair waiting for your grandchildren to show up." He and his wife, who is a nurse, both felt that getting cosmetic procedures to look younger made perfect sense, but younger people getting cosmetic procedures to look more perfect was a dangerous effect of the increased normalization of such procedures.

WIFE: I'm much more sympathetic with an old person getting anti-aging procedures and treatments than a young person trying to look perfect.
HUSBAND: Yeah, everyone thinks they're going to be perfect, like a Barbie or a Ken doll.

WIFE: These people who are having total body makeovers when they're fine. It's not necessary. It's only because the social repercussions are so negative for not being perfect.

This sentiment that it was OK to fight age, but not to become obsessed with perfection, was a fairly common one among baby boomers. One seventy-nine-year-old woman, in a wheelchair, her wrinkle-free and taut face heavily made up, told me that despite having had several breast implants herself over the years, she now regretted wasting money on such "frivolous" procedures, since at her age she really "needed" the money to keep herself from looking "too old." She abruptly ended the interview when I asked her "too old for what?" by saying, "I don't have time for this. I need to get more information about whether I can get another facelift."

It wasn't just baby boomers who saw aging as the problem. A lot of younger patients felt as if they too would work on looking as young as possible for as long as possible. A white woman in her thirties told me that she wouldn't consider Botox yet because needles make her nervous, but "maybe in three years. I don't want to look older. . . . My mom is sixty-two and she's getting a facelift in two weeks and I think that's great. If I need one, I'll get one."

Of course, even many of the people who saw aging as a reason for cosmetic surgery were also critical of our youth-obsessed culture. A fifty-six-year-old white woman who was considering a facelift pointed out that her mother would never have had such a procedure, but today "people are so driven by the media to believe that this is routine. . . . Plastic surgery used to be considered more extreme. People look at it now as if it's a rite of passage, as if outlandish surgical procedures are just part of getting older!"

Like this woman, most patients described America's obsession with youth as driving us to plastic surgery. They also described the media as fueling both our obsession wit our desire for plastic beauty.

It's the Media, Stupid!

Sometimes being a field researcher requires the posing of obvious questions. When I asked cosmetic surgery patients to explain why there has been such an explosion in cosmetic surgery, they looked at me in bafflement, proceeding to explain that, of course, the driving force behind our plastic obsession is the media. A white woman in her thirties observed that "TV's such poison. It's wrecking youth. There are so many commercials for Botox and cosmetic surgery and a week ago she looked like shit and look at her now, after surgery, doesn't she look great?"

A seventy-year-old Black woman sighed when I asked her the question, as if I had insulted her intelligence. Obviously, it all came down to a media-driven quest for perfection:

> People have become so involved in what magazines tell you . . . You're supposed to be perfect. You're supposed to walk on the beach with no love handles. But really we're not all supposed to be perfect. Magazines have all these touch-ups they do on photos so they're not real. . . . It's not reality. . . . The point is that it's projected toward teenagers. Parents have to tell their children, especially girls, with their peer pressure. They're the ones that want to be accepted. [Tell them] "You're good people and feel good about who you are, about being your best. You can't be perfect. You shouldn't feel like you have to be perfect."

An awareness of the role media plays in implanting the desire for cosmetic surgery was common, but also completely beside the point. Plastic surgery still seemed like a potential path to emotional and/or financial well-being, even if that path was strewn with snake oil advertisements offering us perfection and eternal youth.

It's a Bad Thing; I Want It

Wouldn't it be dreary if everyone looked like Britney Spears?
—Potential plastic surgery patient bemoaning
America's growing desire for plastic surgery

A majority of the patients I interviewed expressed some criticism of plastic surgery as a path to a better life.

This [increase in plastic surgery] is probably a bad thing because it's related too often to self-esteem issues. So many issues in the world today. People suffering all over the world. To put your priorities—to make them cosmetic surgery—is so shallow. (Freda)

Some people have gone way too far. . . . Angelina Jolie's lips look great on Angelina Jolie, but not on everyone. . . . It's because we see all these images of teenagers in magazines and stuff. But they're teenagers, not grown women. It's really sad our society is so superficial. (Marta, Latina woman, early thirties)

Olga, a fifty-three-year-old white woman who works in the hospitality industry, expressed a similar sense that the desire for cosmetic surgery was the inevitable result of media pressures: "It's what society pushes on you now. It's everywhere, all these shows, it's like, if you are a bit vulnerable you're going to go for it [get surgery]. I'm in the hospitality business and nine times out of ten the jobs go to the women who look the best. That's just the way it is."

A white woman in her early thirties, who works in real estate, spoke of a friend who had to get surgery to make a good living, but the results were ultimately negative:

Look at silicone; I had a friend who was a bartender on the

beach, you know she had to do it [get implants] to make money and she was making like two grand a week but then [they] burst and she got these lumps in her arms and now she's sick all the time. It ruined her. . . . Those saline ones have to be replaced all the time. It's water. It leaks plus it gets moldy. That can't be good for you. But if I needed them for work . . . I don't know.

Not everyone, however, considered the risks involved in plastic surgery for career advancement. Tina, thirty-two, a large white woman, viewed plastic surgery as the only solution to the roadblocks on her path to success in the IT industry. Tina told me she wants the "bionic package: the tummy tuck, the boob job, the facial rejuvenation." Tina described these potential surgeries as an investment in her career in an industry dominated by men, but also one that rewards the women with the "hottest" bodies.

Gaia, a white woman in her early thirties, put it this way:

Sometimes [plastic surgery] is just *necessary*. Like, I have a friend who had a tummy tuck after . . . having twins. She lost the weight, but the skin stayed loose and she had all these stretch marks. . . . I don't think it's a bad thing. I have a twenty-year-old friend who got a boob job. She felt so good after it that she went from being a bartender to starting school to be a surgical technician. She walked away feeling really good about herself. A lot of people walk out [from cosmetic surgery] feeling great about themselves.

Bill, a fifty-year-old white man, when asked if there is any downside to plastic surgery, responded: "Nah, there's no downside at all when people are feeling better about themselves."

Mia, a forty-something Asian American, also didn't see any downside to cosmetic surgery.

I think it's a good thing, because you wanna look younger because you'll have a happier and better outlook on life. Because when you're old and you have all these wrinkles, you feel depressed. . . . When I look in the mirror and see these sunspots, these bags under my eyes, this stuff I didn't have before, I'm not happy. That's why I want to take care of them. To be happy again.

One young Indian man suggested that it wasn't the media per se, nor the plastic surgery industry, nor even aging baby boomers that had made cosmetic surgery so necessary for happiness. For him, the answer was that American culture had just reached an inevitable "tipping point," Malcolm Gladwell's term for how human behavior is patterned like infectious diseases.[12] Plastic surgery, he said, "used to be in just a few regional pockets in the country, you know, Miami, New York, L.A., but then it spread until it reached a tipping point. Now it's infected us all."

Plastic Doctors

It's not easy to speak with American plastic surgeons—literally; these are some seriously busy people.[13] At the U.S. conferences I attended, between sessions, during lunch and coffee breaks, the surgeons were either busy networking, or on their iPhones or BlackBerrys. My usual method of conducting fieldwork is to walk up and start a conversation, introduce myself, my work, and ask if the person can spare a few minutes to speak with me. This method was effective in Berlin, where doctors from around the world were likely to take a break (and a smoke) without being constantly "plugged in," but it was completely useless in the United States, where plastic surgeons are so thoroughly engaged with their peers and their PDAs that they were rarely vulnerable to the approach of a stranger.

Besides the fact that they're generally seldom alone and unplugged, cosmetic surgeons, especially in the United States, are conspicuous for another reason: they all look more or less the same. From my field notes: *The surgeons are all men and the reporters (on cosmetic surgery) and office people are all women. Everyone is normatively gendered: the men wear well-tailored suits and ties, short hair, wedding rings; the women skirts, heels, cosmetics, long hair.*

A woman who organizes medical conferences told me that cosmetic surgeons are not only more predominantly male as compared with other medical professionals she works with, they're also "better dressed, more charming, better looking." In other words, cosmetic surgeons are much more successful at looking like they're supposed to than I am.

After a day of not being able to speak with many surgeons, I changed my tactic. I put on a dress, some black-seamed hose, some seriously nice shoes, and some makeup. The only way I could get most surgeons to stop what they were doing and look up so that I could say, "Excuse me, may I ask you a few questions?" was by posing as a woman who is engaged in the same aesthetic project as they are. I had to look as if I had spent a lot of time on looking good.

This pose was most certainly not the "real" me. Or to put it in more sociological terms, my "front stage" behavior is generally an attempt to appear casual (even if that casualness is highly produced). I usually wear secondhand T-shirts with Sesame Street characters or local restaurants on them that strike me as "ironic," and jeans. I was once criticized during a job performance review because my hair was "too whatever" (meaning I haven't brushed it regularly since Jimmy Carter was president), and the only cosmetics in my house belong to my daughter. Still, a fieldworker's gotta do what a fieldworker's gotta do. So it is that I began to be a person I wasn't in order to get surgeons to speak with me, often about the person they could transform me into.

Did this "false" self I presented shape the interviews themselves? Were the surgeons more or less likely to answer my "femme fatale" persona honestly? Who knows? What I do know is that they were far more likely to engage with a woman who was obviously engaged in their aesthetic project versus a slightly disheveled professorial type in comfortable shoes. I also know that, for the most part, the surgeons were surprisingly similar in what they thought of their work, their patients, their industry, and what was driving the increasing demand for their services.

Cosmetic Surgeon: Not a Dream Job

Nearly all of the American cosmetic surgeons I interviewed came to cosmetic surgery through reconstructive surgery. In other words, performing boob job after boob job was not their dream in medical school. But soon enough, as the reality of income versus debt level set in, they began to perform more cosmetic surgery. According to the American Medical Association, the average debt of a medical student in 2009 was $154,607, and 79 percent of medical school graduates are at least $100,000 in debt.[14] According to an article in the *New York Times,* plastic surgery and dermatology are now the most competitive subspecialties for medical students, which may indicate that for the next generation of cosmetic surgeons, doing boob jobs *is* their dream job.[15] But even if more students are interested in becoming cosmetic surgeons, most programs still focus on reconstructive surgery.[16] Certainly for the surgeons I interviewed, who were between their mid-thirties and mid-sixties, becoming a cosmetic surgeon was definitely plan B.

As the surgeons acquired a mortgage, a spouse, children, and the inevitable costs of living the American dream, they paid the price by performing more and more cosmetic procedures and fewer reconstructive ones. Jack, a doctor from a southern state, said:

> I couldn't live on just reconstructive work. . . . I didn't realize how quickly I'd have to rely on cosmetic surgery just to make it. I started doing cosmetic stuff in 1994 just to

hedge my practice, but now [aesthetic surgery] is the core. When I went into it, I wanted to help people. I subsequently became a Christian and that's why I haven't stopped reconstructive work.

Kate, a fifty-one-year-old white surgeon from Texas, had a typical trajectory from "serious" surgeon to plastic surgeon.

I was doing reconstructive surgery and a lot of work for cancer patients, but I had kids and my husband is a doctor too and I had to find a way of working and taking care of my kids, so I went into private practice in '97. At first I was able to do reconstructive work still, but now my practice is all aesthetic surgery.

Of course, like most of the surgeons I interviewed, Kate was ultimately happy with her decision. "You know what? I love it. I make the women who come into my office so happy. I give them peace so they can stop thinking about what's bothering them and start having fun with their kids in a bikini."

Another surgeon, this one a sixty-something white man who practiced in Manhattan, also loved performing plastic surgery, because it is "creative" and "artistic." On the other hand, "I have ambivalent feelings myself about all this. My patients think it's a good thing. But I wonder if most of them realize it's all a bunch of fiction." What's fiction? I ask. "This whole thing. This idea that it's going to change their life."

A doctor from North Carolina told me that he is really glad neither his wife nor his teenage daughters want cosmetic surgery, yet it is cosmetic surgery that pays for their privileged lifestyle.

I don't want my wife to get work done. My wife is forty-five years old and 145 pounds and she hates the gym. And she's had three kids. And I think she's beautiful . . . my daughter

lost a lot of weight recently, she went from 115 pounds to
108 and she's been talking a lot about how her breasts disap-
peared, but I don't want her to get implants. It's hard. I'm
talking out of both sides of my mouth . . . My wife and kids
know that our house, our vacations, their school are all paid
for by boob jobs.

The feeling that being a plastic surgeon is "not what I meant
to be doing, but it's a pretty good job" came up in most of the
interviews I had with plastic surgeons from the United States.
Depending on the country, other doctors had a different sense
of what they were doing and why. Most seemed pretty excited
about their work, but some surgeons struggled to place their
work within value systems that would seem to condemn cosmetic surgery. Surgeons who were either very religious or practicing plastic surgery in cultures dominated by a particular
religion (usually fundamentalist Christianity or state-sponsored
Islam) struggled to place their work within the dominant belief
system. Similarly, surgeons who considered themselves feminists had some trouble figuring out whether what they do for a
living is in fact oppressive to women.

Parham, from Iran, told me that although there are only
about 140 cosmetic surgeons in the entire country, aesthetic
surgery is increasingly popular there, especially nose jobs. Two
other surgeons from Iran told me that nose jobs are considered
the height of fashion among urban youth, so much so that they
go out to clubs with plaster on their noses to look as if they just
had a rhinoplasty. About 85 percent of Parham's work in Tehran consists of rhinoplasty: "Everyone in Iran, well, especially
in Tehran, has satellite TV, and around the world no actors or
actresses have bumps in their noses. Even Barbra Streisand had
a nose job. . . . And, after the Revolution, women veiled, so the
face is the only visible part and that makes it even more important." Parham told me that these women want "beautiful noses"

(and, increasingly, anti-aging procedures) for themselves and for their husbands.

A surgeon from the United Arab Emirates told me that rhinoplasty was popular, but not as popular as liposuction. Breast reduction is the third-most-popular procedure in his practice, but breast implants and body contouring are increasing in popularity. His wife, who stood next to him, told me that many women have to be careful about such things since some consider it against Islamic law to show your body unnecessarily to a doctor. The surgeon interrupted her to point out that "God is beautiful and God loves beauty." They both agreed that women were doing it for their husbands.

This sense that plastic surgery was useful for marriage also appeared in some of the interviews with U.S. surgeons, especially those from southern states. A married, white male surgeon from Arkansas said that his patients are 90 percent women, "everyone from hairdressers to Walmart executives' wives." But he will not treat a woman who is planning on getting a divorce.

> I'm a very conservative plastic surgeon. I won't operate on everyone. If someone is going through a major life change I tell them they should hold off . . . I often see women in two-income couples and she is paying with her money and I say I won't do it till you talk to your husband about this . . . If I thought a woman were doing it to leave her husband, I wouldn't help. Or strippers . . . I wouldn't make a breast so big it stuck outside of the rib cage . . . or transsexual surgery. I don't do penile implants or things like that. I don't do any kind of surgery that's abnormal or making them different from the norm . . . I have to think about it. I pray with patients before I operate.

Although this particular surgeon had a more defined sense of morally right and morally wrong cosmetic surgery than most,

doctors from Georgia, Alabama, and both North and South Carolina told me that they had questions on their intake forms about
changes in marital status and tried to discourage women who
were either considering a divorce or getting one from having too
much work done. Usually the surgeons felt not just that it was
unethical to aid and abet a divorce, but that it would be a waste of
money for the woman. For instance, a doctor from a southern state
told me that when he sees a client who is about to get a divorce:

> I try to talk her down a bit. I say, "Let's not do everything
> right now." Maybe do a little face rejuvenation. Something
> noninvasive. Because they're going to go to the bar and it's
> going to be filled with twenty-year-olds and, because that
> was the last time they were dating, they want to look twenty
> and it's filled with all these guys in their twenties and they're
> not interested in them but in the twenty-year-old girls, and
> maybe there's a few older men, but they're also looking for
> twenty-year-old girls . . . I know these women will just leave
> my office and go to the surgeon down the street, but I'm still
> a doctor and I have to treat the whole person. My first rule is
> to do no harm.

Many of the southern doctors talked about being Christian
and believing that the work they do is part of that Christian mission. One evangelical Christian surgeon I interviewed, when I
asked what Jesus would think of cosmetic surgery, responded:
"Jesus's first miracle was to turn water into wine. Isn't that what
I do every day?" This man was not alone in believing that Jesus,
were he here today, would be a plastic surgeon. One presenter at
the international conference in Berlin said that plastic surgeons
represent "the moment of transfiguration when Christ's body is
made whole again. Plastic surgery can erase the pain of stigmata."
    Feminism presented an equally difficult belief system for
some plastic surgeons. An English surgeon, a white woman in

her thirties who identified herself as a feminist, told me that she believed we were experiencing a third wave of feminism. "Hopefully things are turning the other way now. Hopefully we'll go back the other way and actually oppose women being so thin, picking models who are so thin. And these magazines are always showing that women should be thin with big boobs."

Another white, female surgeon, this one in her fifties and from a southern state in the U.S., expressed a similar desire for an end to her thriving practice in cosmetic procedures. "Maybe people will stop when they realize it's more important to save the earth. Maybe they'll go organic or all natural . . . Maybe they'll learn it's more important to be at peace on the inside than it is to look good."

David, a plastic surgeon from New Zealand, made an extremely good living doing boob jobs. The disconnect between his work and his feminist values, however, weighed on him. Eventually he decided that the inherent "woman-hating" of boob jobs, plus the absolute boredom of doing what he considered a ridiculously easy procedure, were just not in line with who he wanted to be. David closed his lucrative private practice and went back to work for a public hospital, doing reconstructive work.

It's the Same Everywhere, but It's Different Here

Many plastic surgeons from countries with universal healthcare systems were still doing quite a bit of reconstructive work. A young (thirty-four-year-old) Austrian surgeon told me that he mostly does breast reductions, not augmentations. "We have a different body culture here. Of course if there's a congenital deformity or cancer, we'll reconstruct and even augment the breast, but most Austrians consider the American [cosmetic surgery] too extreme."

Surgeons from a variety of European countries agreed that there are huge differences between European and American cosmetic surgery practices. A young French surgeon tells me: "In France we're not allowed to perform these extreme makeovers.

In America a woman wants to be seen as having work done. If people can't see she's had a facelift, she'll be disappointed. She wants people to see she's had her breasts done."

A surgeon from Frankfurt told me that the German government has really stepped up its efforts to regulate the cosmetic surgery industry there. "So for instance we're not allowed to show before and after photos in our ads anymore. The government thinks people are so stupid that they cannot think for themselves. They say they're doing it to protect the patient . . . but in America . . . anything goes."

A woman who practices in London described her work at a public hospital as consisting of tummy tucks, eyelid lifts, and breast reductions because the National Health Service will pay for them. The NHS will also pay for breast augmentation if a psychiatrist determines it "necessary," as well as transsexual surgery and any aesthetic procedures, like rhinoplasty, that might help a person pass in their chosen gender.

Although most western Europeans saw their cosmetic surgery industry as starkly different from the American one, most South Americans saw what they do as similar to that of the United States' and different from Europe's. Marta, a forty-three-year-old surgeon from Chile, emphasized that the Americas are similar in their cosmetic practices.

> People from the Americas—North and South—are different from the Europeans. For Europeans, wrinkles are a part of life. But in the Americas we want to be younger. In Europe everything is already old; everything's done. It's over. They work less. They're through. Is this evolution forward or are they going back? People [in Europe] just want to be what they are. . . . In Europe plastic surgery is still done very discreetly. Whenever I come [to Europe] and people find out what I do, they [say] "Oh no, we should be getting old with dignity" and then the next day they quietly come to me and ask me for my advice.

A fortysomething surgeon who has an aesthetic and reconstructive practice in Columbia argued that although his practice
is similar to that of doctors in the United States, the two cultures are starkly different:

> [In the United States] in order to have good work you have
> to look young and healthy. Also, you treat old people...
> They're almost thrown away [in the United States]. It's dif-
> ferent in Columbia because the family is still very close. But
> when I lived here in New York I said hello to an old woman,
> a neighbor, one day, and she stopped and nearly cried. No
> one had spoken to her for a month. It's as if old people here
> are ghosts. No wonder people feel they have to look young.

A sixty-eight-year-old female surgeon from Delhi, India,
told me that her country is different from both the United
States and Europe in the amount of cosmetic procedures performed: "In the U.S., a plastic surgeon does ninety percent
aesthetic surgery, in Britain about fifty percent of their practice, and in India only about ten percent of plastic surgery is
aesthetic and the rest is reconstructive. [This is because] to a
beggar, plastic surgery has no meaning. They're interested in
food, not a facelift."

She, however, practices only aesthetic surgery. She has been
doing facelifts for thirty-two years and she thinks the reasons
for anti-aging surgery are the same everywhere: "People want to
look good. Often the husband is looking to this side and that...
A fifty-five-year-old man is always young and dashing; a fifty-
five-year-old woman is old and haggard."

If plastic surgeons disagreed over whether national cultures
shaped their practices, they did agree on the causes for the nearly
universal increase in the demand for cosmetic surgery: fashion,
media and technology.

Technology, TV, and Thongs
TECHNOLOGY
Sitting in an air-conditioned lecture hall at the Mandalay Bay Resort in Las Vegas, I dutifully write down all the "technological breakthroughs" that are supposedly driving the industry. Boob jobs that use stem cells from pigs and temporary boob jobs with fillers and other elixirs of youth and beauty are touted as the "next big thing." I leave the lecture hall and interview a surgeon (white, male, sixty-three) from the Bay Area who has the next big thing in the treatment of cellulite (but it's a secret for now) and it, too, will revolutionize the industry. Many of the surgeons I interviewed and a majority of the vendors saw advances in technology as the number one reason cosmetic surgery is so increasingly necessary.

Brad, a fifty-year-old surgeon from Connecticut, believed that technology is driving the demand.

> People are living longer and they're taking care of themselves and you look in the mirror and want to look as good on the outside as you feel . . . There's the technology out there that allows people to change and improve and it's minimally invasive. I did some myself . . . I got to a point after my daughter graduated from high school last year and I was looking at photos and saw this guy who looked familiar with gray hair and a baggy neck and I realized that was me! That's what I looked like. And that just wasn't my body image. So I did some laser things. I tightened it all up a bit.

Another fifty-something, white male surgeon, this one from Alabama, tells me that the new and improved silicone implants and the new and improved "through-the-belly-button" implantation of them means he can do a boob job in under fifteen minutes. In a typical Fordist model of production, he can get everything cheaper because he does such a huge volume, thereby passing the

savings on to consumers, who are that much more likely to consider implants given how inexpensive he can make them.

Vendors of cosmetic surgery products, who tended to be far
more openly cynical about the industry than their surgical comrades, saw the products they represented as creating demand.
One vendor told me that demand for cosmetic surgery is driven
by "a cycle of innovation. Something new is invented. This
drives the fervor. The fervor drives these [consumers] to want
these things. Then these things drive innovation. But it's not
just fervor. It's dementia!"

In other words, vendors saw the technologies they represent as
driving demand, but they also often believed that was a bad thing.
One vendor told me he wanted to bring his young children to the
plastic surgery conference so he could say to them: "See this. This
is everything that's wrong with this culture. So grow up to do
something worthwhile with your life. Do not end up like this."

TV

Like their patients, a lot of surgeons saw the media as fueling their
industry. For some this was a bad thing; for others it was good
news. A Southern-U.S., white male surgeon had this to say:

> My patients are always quoting *Dr. 90210*. My [all-female]
> staff too. Look, they had an episode on G-spot augmentation
> in April. Every single woman on my staff said she wanted to
> do it. So we did two on employees and it WORKS! It makes
> it so you can feel the G-spot without rear entry by placing
> the tip of the penis in the right place. We do this by inflat-
> ing the vaginal canal . . . These shows definitely affect my
> practice. We always get a lot of traffic the next day. And even
> bad news increases business. Like the [near] death of that
> rapper's wife? Because people start talking and then girls
> who've had some work done will say, "I love my breast aug-
> mentations," and that just increases business.

A California breast-implant vendor, a Latino man in his thirties, also thought it was media-driven, but in very culturally specific ways.

> We live in an aesthetic-driven society, and a certain amount of it is cultural, the media. But look around you [indicating a nearly all-white crowd in Manhattan].
> It really depends what neighborhood you're from. How many Black women do this? They're just more grounded. . . . It's mostly a white woman thing, although the Asian population is buying in too. . . .
> The States are a hyper-individualistic place. It's always, How's my job? What kind of car am I driving? How does my butt look? Never, How's my neighbor doing? But I have no pity for them. Turn it off dude! Turn the TV off, for Christ's sake!

A New York State surgeon was so frustrated with the influence that reality TV has on his patients that he waxed poetic in a manner not so different from postmodern philosopher Michel Foucault. "My patients are so influenced by the media. They all want to look like twelve-year-old boys. . . . People are . . . so subjected [by the media] that they've lost their own subjectivity."

Surgeons from around the world agreed that Hollywood is increasing the demand for cosmetic surgery. A thirty-five-year-old surgeon from South Korea said that there everyone wants eyelid surgery (creating a "double lid") because "everyone wants to look like American movie stars." An Iranian surgeon said that Disney made the "Persian nose a problem." Surgeons from Armenia, France, Germany, Estonia, and England all told me that when cosmetic surgery shows like *Dr. 90210* and *Extreme Makeover* air, their offices are inundated with new patients the next day. A surgeon from Colombia said that Hollywood shows definitely inspire people to come into his office. "Some of my colleagues th[

shows are positive, like propaganda. And definitely we get more patients. But these shows distort reality by presenting aesthetic surgery as if it were the same as getting a haircut. And that's a risky strategy."

A surgeon from Germany told me that patients often bring in photographs of Hollywood celebrities and say, "Make me look like that." Like the patients, surgeons understood that "it's the media, stupid!" Unlike many of their patients, however, they also saw fashion, the shape and cut of the clothes we wear, as creating the desire to reshape our bodies.

THONGS

According to a white American surgeon in her fifties, plastic surgery is the inevitable outcome of clothes that make nearly everyone look as if they're overweight.

> It's the fashion. It's clothes. These low-cut jeans. I have to do the abdominoplasty lower and lower. You have to cut more, but I tell them to bring in a bikini or jeans and we work from there. But they're so low-cut that anyone would look bad in them. I always say those jeans have brought more business my way than anything. And the clothes they work out in. It's not T-shirts. They wear these tops that are basically bras and tight bottoms and it brings them into my office.

A white surgeon from a southern state whose wife had recently had breast implants told me: "I wish my wife hadn't done it. But with fashion the way it is today, she just couldn't get clothes to fit. Couldn't find a bathing suit. The breasts are just way more visible. Same with flat stomachs. The clothes just emphasize those parts of it more."

Another white, male surgeon, this one forty-three and from a beach community in Long Island, said that the fact that "people spend all summer on the boat means they want to look good. Bikinis. So there's a lot of gym work. A lot of cosmetic work."

Many surgeons suggested that the rise in vaginoplasty was directly related to the removal of pubic hair. A white male surgeon from a Southern state asked: "Do you really think anyone would care if they still had their pubic hair? Who would even notice? And it's the same with bigger breasts and flat stomach. It's because clothes emphasize it more."

In other words, it was technology, TV, and thongs driving the increased demand for cosmetic surgery. For surgeons, the increasing demand for cosmetic surgery was most certainly *not* the result of the surgeons' actions themselves. In fact, surgeons went out of their way to paint themselves as "just meeting customers' demands." Even as they poked at my face and announced what was wrong and what was needed, surgeons saw themselves as just doing their jobs, answering demands produced outside of their offices by a culture over which they had no control.

Our Industry Is Innocent

No surgeons were willing to say that it was the surgeons themselves who implanted the desire for surgery in their patients. An Indian American surgeon in his early thirties who had recently started a practice in aesthetic procedures thought that it would be much better if the demand for cosmetic procedures would just go away. Still, he pointed out, if he didn't do it, someone else would. To emphasize this point, he told me a story about a woman who was seven months pregnant who came into his office demanding Botox because her husband told her she looked tired. He wisely informed her that she couldn't do Botox during pregnancy, that "she should stop worrying about looking good and bring the baby into the world healthy . . . because if she hurts her baby, she will never forgive herself. That's a lifetime. Not the short-term effects of pregnancy on her face."

The woman, of course, went to the aesthetic spa down the

street, a place with no direct medical supervision, and had it done anyway. "What can you do?" he asked, shrugging his shoulders.

Yet, cosmetic surgeons don't just respond to the demand to fix women's bodies. As historian Elizabeth Haiken points out, surgeons play an active role in creating the desire for cosmetic surgery. Such desire isn't just the result of cultural messages, but

> is created each day in each surgeon's office during the series of exchanges during which patients' requests fit, or not, with what a surgeon believes to be appropriate and desirable. Surgeons who over the course of the century have agreed with their patients that Jewish noses should be made smaller, that Asian eyes should be made to open wider; that lines and wrinkles are ugly and who have then acted on those convictions have played a role commensurate with the flood of perfect images that inspired the initial inquiries.[17]

Many patients told me they initially went to the plastic surgeons hoping they would tell them "there's nothing wrong" with them. Instead they heard a list of what was wrong and what could be done to fix it. So did I. The following is a partial list of what I was told by surgeons while researching this book:

> *You need a midface lift. . . . You need a facelift. . . . Have you ever considered a nose job?. . . Breast implants and a lift would help with your ptosis and loss of volume. . . . Breast implants would make you look less boyish. . . . Have you considered butt implants?. . . Nasolabial fillers?. . . An eyelid lift. Maybe some lipo . . . You should get: Juvéderm, Botox, lip implants, microdermabrasion. . . . You need a drink.*

This last need, a drink, was from a woman at a cocktail party for female plastic surgeons. I had snuck in, thinking I might "pass" as one of them, and I did. In truth, a room full of women cosmetic surgeons doesn't look that different from a gathering of sociologists; slightly better dressed, perhaps, but just as likely to be in "need' of a haircut, dye job, good night's sleep, and a drink as the rest of us. One of the women there told me that as a cosmetic surgeon she felt like she "ought" to at least get Botox regularly, but "who has the time? I have two kids, and a husband, and I can't even find time to go get my hair cut and dyed regularly, let alone worry about how old I look."

I nodded in agreement, the double burden of being both a professional and a woman weighing heavily on us both. Then she leaned in for a closer look and I waited to hear her advice on what I should do. Which part of my body would inspire her to insist I get it fixed?

"You know what you need? A drink. Me too."

As she handed me a glass of white wine, she clinked my glass and we toasted our careers and our children. She didn't even mention my nasolabial folds or her own sagging jaw line, and at that moment I thought: perhaps we can escape plastic? I had a real feeling of hope and solidarity with this woman, this plastic surgeon who described her work as "tummy tucks and boob jobs" on women who left their own careers to be stay-at-home wives in a wealthy suburb of a southern American city. We were, in many ways, completely different, and yet I could see that we were also more or less living fairly similar lives. We drank our wine and talked shop about male-dominated careers, the difficulties of raising children who care about more than how they look, and the way mass media controls us all. Then I went back to my room and turned on the TV. My hope for a plastic-free future seemed ridiculously naive in the glare of the TV set. As I explore in the next two chapters, we are all, each and every one of us—the plastic surgeon and the professor—trapped in a visual culture that increasingly demands that we go under the knife.

PART II

Boob Jobs and Credit Cards

CHAPTER 4

Learning to Be Plastic
Magazines, TV, and Other Cultural Scripts

Turning forty is considered a problem in our culture. Even poet Maya Angelou, in her poem "On Reaching Forty," suggests that those who survive forty best "have the inborn wisdom and grace and are clever enough to die at thirty-nine."[1] This problem is especially vexing for women, since the forties mark the beginning of the end, the last decade in which we can legitimately be considered objects of sexual desire. When pop superstar Madonna was about to turn fifty, a *Vanity Fair* reporter wrote: "Madonna is turning 50 in August. Madonna made her fortune selling sex— what will she sell when the thought of sex with Madonna seems like a fetish?"[2] Finding a fifty-year-old woman sexually attractive is apparently as unusual as wanting to copulate with a shoe. Women of a certain age are a fetish; not a legitimate object of desire. These things are said about Madonna, whose body and face, thanks to an obsessive workout routine as well as cosmetic interventions, are still "perfect."

The revulsion to Madonna as a sexual being haunted me when I turned forty. Unlike Madonna's decade-older body, my forty-year-old body collapsed. I went from being extremely athletic to having a bad knee to having knee surgery. I lay on the couch for weeks, on too many painkillers to do much but read and watch television. I flipped through women's and pop culture magazines and watched TV shows about plastic surgery. It was like trying to cure the chicken pox by introducing HIV into the organism. I went from feeling a slight sense of foreboding about the ugliness of an aging body to a full-blown disgust at every part of my body, but especially those parts that marked me as "aged." The slight sagging of my too-small breasts, the lines of my nasolabial folds, the stretch marks on my stomach from two pregnancies floated through my drug-addled brain as signs of my damnation to the cursed state of undesirable.

After I recovered, I went back to ignoring TV and pop culture magazines. My knee healed. My body returned to its pre-forty routines. Slowly, I started to pay less attention to my collapsing, disgusting, revolting body. The problem of turning forty faded, still there, but less acute, like a body that has healed itself of the pox, but is still infected with a potentially deadly virus. Looking back on my initiation into being a "certain age," I realize that what infected me was *ordinary ugliness.* Ordinary ugliness is what we all experience: stretch marks, cellulite, wrinkles, the downward pull of gravity, the realization that our bodies are not and can never really be perfect. Ordinary ugliness is part of a set of beliefs that infect all of us, no matter how hard we try to avoid them. The next two chapters explore some of the cultural scripts that tell us that ordinary bodies, especially ordinary, middle-aged female bodies, are ugly, and the only way to live in them is to alter them with cosmetic procedures.

The Plastic Ideological Complex

> *My abiding life philosophy is plain: In our appearance-centric society, beauty is a huge factor in everyone's professional and emotional success—for good or ill, it's the way things are; accept it or go live under a rock.*
>
> — JOAN RIVERS

In her apologia for cosmetic surgery, *Men Are Stupid . . . And They Like Big Boobs,* Joan Rivers tells us that cosmetic surgery is an unavoidable part of modern life.[3] She would know. Rivers herself has become a symbol of the perfectly smooth, perfectly produced septuagenarian. Rivers had a nose job in college, her first facelift in her early forties, and has continued with a variety

of nips and tucks and monthly nonsurgical cosmetic "mainte-
nance." The result is startling. Rivers looks like she's half her
age. Her utterly smooth face—that barely moves—is like a
mask of beauty. This beauty has the slightly blurred edge of one
too many procedures. There is a nearly imperceptible difference
between the left and the right eyes, the result, no doubt, of the
endless battle against time and gravity. And yet, there is no de-
nying that Rivers does not look at all like the old woman she is.

But Rivers is a TV star. TV and movie stars have always
utilized the miracles of cosmetic surgery to look good in the
two-dimensional spaces they inhabit. How did the rest of us
learn to desire a perfectly plastic body? How did ordinary
women and men with ordinary lives and ordinary bodies learn
that they need plastic? The answer: the *plastic ideological complex,* a set of cultural texts that are both highly contested and
yet tightly on message. It is itself so ubiquitous that it might
even be described as hegemonic. In other words, the "need" for
cosmetic procedures is impossible to avoid. Through advertising and TV shows, movies and magazines, we learn to want
cosmetic intervention in our aging faces and imperfect bodies.
This need is now so firmly implanted in our cultural psyche that
it has become "common sense" to embrace cosmetic procedures.
Why wouldn't we want to look more beautiful, younger, thinner, more feminine, better? The question is no longer will you
have plastic surgery, but when.

Accept plastic beauty or go live under a rock. Rivers isn't
just joking; she's also doing the serious work of enacting the
ideology of plastic, an ideology that we can no longer avoid.
Even if we did live under a rock, whenever we crawled out from
underneath it, we would be assaulted by images of perfectly
plastic beauty on billboards and the sides of buses and on TV
and in movies and even the nightly news. And then there are
those damn magazine racks, an unavoidable gauntlet of Dos!
and Don'ts! that must be passed through each and every time

we buy our food. "Kelly Ripa Doesn't Rule Out Plastic Surgery" and "Jessica Simpson: I'd Get Plastic Surgery" and "Liv Tyler 'Definitely' Wants Plastic Surgery." These recent headlines from *People* magazine tell us that plastic surgery is what the stars do, and who doesn't want to be like the stars?

That's how plastic surgery arrives as "the answer" for an increasing number of Americans, especially women. The plastic ideological complex produces plastic propaganda to demand that we look a certain way or go under the knife. The propaganda instructs us on what is necessary to be fully human, or at least fully female. Sociologists call this instruction a cultural script. Cultural scripts give us our lines, our cues, our costumes, and our setting. How well we enact a particular script varies from individual to individual and group to group. Joan Rivers is a brilliant actor of plastic beauty; I can barely stumble through my lines. Our actions are shaped by plastic propaganda, but not fully determined by them. Some of us, like Joan Rivers, will follow the scripts carefully; others, on the fringes of society, will resist and organize their lives against these scripts. These are the women who will allow their beards to grow in, not shave their legs, and never dye their hair. The vast majority of us will both follow *and* resist. We just hope we can muddle through the performance of beauty without anything too embarrassing happening. We are not looking for a standing ovation for our plastic beauty; but we don't want to have rotten fruit thrown at us for being horrendous social actors either.

The Beauty Industry

Performing plastic melts into other cultural scripts, like the beauty and diet industries and self-improvement. As a variety of scholars have pointed out, the beauty and diet industries sell American women on the "body project," the idea that they must spend most of their resources on their looks or fail. Because the body project relies on selling us more and more, it has to make us feel worse and worse. In other words, the requirements of beauty only ever go up, not down.

In my own family, my grandmother, who was born at the end of the nineteenth century, never dyed her hair or wore lipstick. For my grandmother, actresses and prostitutes cared about how they looked; "ordinary" women were good mothers and wives. My mother, who was born in the 1920s, began to care about the way she looked in her late teens, dyed her hair, dieted, and wore lipstick for the first few decades of her adult life. Like most women of her generation, my mother stopped caring about how she looked after her children were born. By late middle age, my mother believed it was acceptable to "let herself go." My mother had a sister who refused to stop working on her body. This sister continued to wear high heels, cover her face in a heavy layer of foundation and aqua blue eye shadow, and dye her huge bee-hive blond well into her sixties. My mother considered this behavior morally suspect. Continued engagement in beauty was a sure sign of wanting to go out with other women's husbands, or worse. I wonder what my mother, if she were alive, would think of me or of her granddaughters. I myself spend countless hours trying to maintain the same body in my forties that I had in my twenties. Even after giving birth to my daughters, I feel that I must at least try. I don't know at what age I can stop dying my hair or working out, but it's definitely not anytime soon, if ever. My daughters began beauty work—shaving and cosmetics and hair dying—before puberty and will no doubt still be engaged in this work when they're very old women.

Historian Joan Jacobs Brumberg provides concrete proof that the body project is getting bigger, not smaller, as consumer capitalism makes us work on previously unheard of problems. In *The Body Project: An Intimate History of American Girls,* Brumberg reads the journals of young women over the course of a century to illustrate how what is expected of them only increases over time. "Girls today," Brumberg argues, "make the body into an all-consuming project in ways young women of the past did not." Although young women a century ago were both self-conscious and always judged by community standards, it was behavior more than beauty that set the standard. Beauty imperatives for girls in the nineteenth century were kept in check by consideration of moral character.

> Many parents tried to limit their daughters' interest in superficial things, such as hairdos, dresses, or the size of their waists, because character was considered more important than beauty by both parents and the community. And character was built on attention to self-control, service to others, and belief in God—not on attention to one's own, highly individualistic body project.[4]

When I tell my daughters to worry about their character, not their hair or the size of their breasts, they laugh at how ridiculously out of touch I am with the reality of middle-school life in the twenty-first century.

Not only do the requirements of the body project increase over time, but the standards of beauty are also constantly shifting. What is beautiful today is not what was beautiful in my time. Middle-school girls today pluck and shape their eyebrows into thin arches; in my time we all wanted the thick eyebrows of Brooke Shields. At times small breasts have been the gold standard, at others an ample bosom. Sometimes large, heavy hips and legs are the norm, at others thin legs and narrow hips. I have a book from 1902 called *The Body Beautiful: Common Sense Ideas on Health and Beauty without Medicine* by Nannette Magruder Pratt. The book contains advice on how to get stronger, fatter (apparently you could be too thin), and have regular bowel movements. Most of the advice centers on dress reform. "Tight-lacing brings about a dreadful condition of all of the vital organs," warns Pratt.[5] The book contains a series of photographs of women, free of corsets, engaged in a variety of exercises to expand their lungs or strengthen their legs. The women are in their thirties, with no cosmetics or eyebrow plucking visible on their faces. Their bodies are small-waisted, but curvaceous. When I showed the photographs of these turn-of-the-century beauties to my teenage daughter, she said, "Oh, they're so ugly. And fat." Beauty one hundred years ago is "ugly" and "fat" today. I'm guessing that by 1902 standards, when women were encouraged to be healthy, but also kind and good at needlepoint, Joan Rivers would be considered a hideous monster.

The Self-Help Industry

In addition to the body project, there is also a more specifically American project of "self-improvement," the idea that our bodies and psyches are infinitely malleable and can always be made better. This deep-seated sense that we can always improve ourselves is at the center of what it means to be an American. *Work hard and you'll succeed. Try, try, and try again. What doesn't kill us, makes us stronger.* This work for work's sake is what sociologist Max Weber called the "Protestant ethic." In his seminal 1905 book *The Protestant Ethic and the Spirit of Capitalism,* Weber argued that capitalism took off in America because of our culture, not our structure. In other words, the necessary elements of capitalism were in place long before the Industrial Revolution. Money, exchange, trade routes, and machines existed in China and Venice, among other places, centuries before manufacturing took off in the New World. The reason that capitalism didn't take off in these places is because the spirit of the time, the zeitgeist, did not move people to invest all their energy into work and then reinvest any and all profit into making more profit. The Protestant sects that thrived on American soil believed it was not just good, but godly, to devote one's life to industry and profit. This spirit made people work harder. Although over time the American work ethic lost its religious roots, the idea that being a good person was being a financially successful person never went away. And so we work and work and work to make our lives and our bodies better.[6]

In an interesting twist, the American work ethic was then transformed into the self-help industry. It became important not just to work hard to make money, but also to work hard to make ourselves "better" people. This desire for self-improvement was then translated into a moneymaking opportunity by a variety of self-help gurus, from Sigmund Freud's psychoanalysis to Suzanne Somers's ThighMaster. As Micki McGee puts it in *Self-Help, Inc.,* "The ideal of self-invention has long infused American culture with a sense of endless possibility."[7] The beauty and diet industry are part of the self-help spirit of America. Even an ugly gal can look better with the right lipstick. If your hair is gray, dye it and look younger. If you don't have a perfect body, diet and go to the gym—or pay a visit to a plastic surgeon.

But this isn't just about the middle-aged white women who are the most likely to go under the knife. It's about all of us. Consumer capitalism has to sell us stuff—that's its purpose—and so it sells us a better version of ourselves. Pay a therapist in order to be more mentally stable; pay a financial adviser in order to become more fiscally sound. For some of us, an increasing number of us, the way to become better is to become more beautiful. Beauty used to be for adult women, then girls. Now, beauty is something many men, particularly young men of the professional classes, must consider. A look at a magazine like *Men's Health* reveals just how many products must be bought and grooming practices engaged in to be a desirable man. How can you turn that gut into a six-pack? What about whiter teeth? Thinning hair: what should you do? Because capitalist systems seek to constantly increase profit, beauty capitalism must constantly invent new forms of beauty and new problems to be solved with new products. To keep beauty profitable, our bodies must be colonized as if they were foreign lands. In this way, beauty can create new markets and extract more wealth.

According to feminist theorist Susan Bordo, we have reached
a point in time where we are ruled by an ideology that tells us
that there is no limit to how much we can improve and transform our bodies. "We now have . . . cultural plastic . . . we
now have ourselves, the master sculptor of that plastic."[8] Bordo's
cultural plastic marks our current historical moment as unprecedented in human history. It's not unusual that we have standards of beauty. What's unusual is that we believe ourselves to
be masters of that beauty, to be in charge of our own physical
manifestation, to be our own gods. It is that belief in the plastic nature of our bodies, their infinite ability to improve and
change shape, that is exploited for profit and transmitted primarily through visual media. We learn what we need to buy and
also *why* we need to buy it primarily through imitating what we
are taught to see as beautiful. In other words, the implantation
of surgical desires started with the birth of consumer capitalism and its twin, visual culture, and together they produced the
plastic ideological complex.

What follows is an exploration of how we learn to need plastic today. My method for documenting the plastic ideological
complex is simple. I listened to what the consumers of cosmetic
surgery were saying. What did they read or watch or consume
that implanted a desire for cosmetic surgery? Then I looked
around myself and asked: If I had just arrived in our time and
place with no knowledge of it, let's say I had just crawled out
from under a rock, how would I know that certain bodies need
surgery? How would I learn to desire plastic surgery? The plastic ideological complex comes in a variety of forms: newspapers,
books, art, movies, TV shows, magazines, newspapers. These
representations of plastic beauty are not all the same. Some are
simply propaganda for plastic; others take a more ambivalent
approach to plastic beauty. All of the messages are complicated
by things like class, race, and sexuality.[9] Yet despite the inner
contradictions of these texts, they are all in agreement on one
thing: cosmetic surgery is a normal part of beauty, and beauty

requires consumption. This doesn't mean that the women and men who consume these scripts of plastic immediately run out to a plastic surgeon's office. What it does mean is that these are the cultural scripts and ideal forms that have the most "prestige," and therefore we are expected to imitate them. Who we most want to be is a series of images we once saw on-screen or in the pages of magazines.

Plastic Magazines: *O* the *Allure* of *New Beauty*

It looks like plastic surgery to me because it's so tight and plastic-y.

—*ALLURE* READER, on why singer Fergie
looks so hot in the magazine's photos of her

I will be the first to tell you if I ever have plastic surgery.
—OPRAH WINFREY, to her audience

Nearly all magazines that are about "women," "health," or "entertainment" are part of the plastic ideological complex. Plastic surgery peeps out from celebrity magazines like *Us* and *People,* with their regular articles on "who did what" and "who denies it." The plastic ideological complex is visible in tabloids like the *National Enquirer* with their "worst plastic surgery ever" photos. Among magazines aimed at women, many of the beauty and fashion magazines, such as *Cosmopolitan* and even *Ladies' Home Journal,* have regular articles on Botox or liposuction. A recent study looking at how women's magazines write about cosmetic surgery found that these magazines consistently portray cosmetic surgery as part of a normal beauty regimen, akin to diet and exercise.[10]

I chose to look at three magazines: *O, Allure,* and *New Beauty.* Each of these magazines has a slightly different demographic and a slightly different message, but all three of them are selling a particular form of beauty that increasingly requires medical intervention. *O* magazine is the lifestyle magazine for Oprah's audience: female, middle-aged, and primarily white (although at 25 percent African American readers, slightly less white than the other magazines). The median age of the *O* reader is 45.9; she is just as likely to be single or divorced as married, but her household income, at a median of $71,000, is well above the national average.[11] *Allure* is important to the culture of plastic because it is, according to Joan Kron, one of its senior editors, the only magazine of its kind that has a full-time reporter covering the cosmetic surgery industry.[12] It is also, at least according to its mission statement, "the only magazine devoted to beauty . . . *Allure* investigates and celebrates beauty and fashion with objectivity and candor, and places appearance in a larger cultural context."[13] *Allure* is aimed at the twenty-five- to forty-five-year-old woman. The *Allure* reader is married and college-educated. She is also primarily white and middle class. *New Beauty,* according to its publisher, is meant to reach everyone from the wealthy woman who can afford cosmetic surgery to the secretary who will give anything and everything for a new look. I chose to include *New Beauty* because it is the only magazine specifically about plastic beauty—that's the "new" part. *New Beauty* is also new in other ways: it uses an editorial board made up of cosmetic surgeons, it has regional editions with pages of contact information for nearby surgeons, and its advertising-to-content ratio is the highest in the magazine world.[14] All three of these magazines have circulations that reach hundreds of thousands of readers. More importantly, all three of the magazines are easily available. You can buy them at your local grocery store, your local bookstore, even your local home-improvement store.

O is not just about beauty and health, but life with a capital *L*. The magazine offers articles on relationships, money, career, and even politics, the environment, and poverty. Despite the serious nature of much of *O*'s content, the magazine also instructs its readers on what to wear, what makeup they need, and a variety of cosmetic procedures. Like Oprah herself, *O* is a unique blend of the spiritual and the material. As religious studies professor Kathryn Lofton points out, "There is something religious about Oprah Winfrey." This religiosity is evident in *O* magazine, where "every product of Winfrey's empire, combines . . . inner awakening with . . . exuberant consumerism."[15] Plastic beauty constitutes part of the exuberant consumption of *O* magazine.

Starting in March 2004, *O* magazine began to feature an average of one article per issue on cosmetic procedures that can improve your life.[16] For instance, July 2007 contains an article on cosmetic dentistry called "Whiter! Straighter! Brighter!" while February 2009 had an article about using stem cells to grow bigger breasts called "A Tuck Here, A Plump There." Slightly less than 10 percent of the advertisements in *O* are for cosmetic enhancements or anti-aging products: teeth-whitening products, anti-aging skin creams, as well as a few for Botox and Juvéderm. The Juvéderm ad showcases a young white woman with parentheses drawn where her nasolabial folds would be if she were ten years older. The slogan is: "Parentheses have a place but not on your face." Further down, the ad tells us that skin injected with Juvéderm is "so smooth and natural, everyone will notice (but no one will know)." The earliest Botox ads I found, beginning in 2004, feature a white woman and an invitation to her twenty-fifth high school reunion with the tag line, "Still waiting for the right time to ask your doctor about Botox Cosmetic?" A more recent Botox ad plays on the nearly religious capitalism of the Oprah empire. The ad features a young Black woman smiling, with the tagline, "It's all about freedom of expression . . . Ask your doctor about BOTOX cosmetic."

If *O* readers are interested in uplifting notions like "freedom of expression," *Allure* readers are more interested in beauty, fashion, and celebrity.[17] *Allure* readers reject the spirituality of *O* and instead embrace a constant state of panic that they might age. Nearly all of the articles about clothes, cosmetics, hairstyles, and fashion are presented as making the reader younger. Learn "Ten Beauty Mistakes That Add Ten Years" or "Get Youthful Skin: 12 Anti-Aging Skin Tricks" or "10 Hairstyles that Make You Look 10 Years Younger." But we also learn that cosmetic procedures are a necessary part of being beautiful, with articles like "The Botox of Tomorrow: Five Cutting-Edge Treatments." Even with the economic downturn, *Allure* readers must continue to look perfectly smooth and wrinkle-free. However, the perfect look can be achieved for less money by cutting some corners, like wearing bangs so no one can see your (wrinkled) forehead. In other words, even if you're broke, you "must" continue to get Botox in the visible part of your face, but you could let your covered-up forehead go to the dogs, since no one but you will see it.[18]

A regular *Allure* feature, "Clock Stoppers," advises women to look out for age spots, use makeup to look younger, and consider cosmetic intervention long before they are even middle-aged. In one "Clock Stoppers," a cosmetic surgeon warns young women to limit facial expression, since it will lead to lines in the face.

> Even among women in their 20s and 30s, when you grimace a lot, you need to break the habit. By disabling the muscles temporarily with Botox, you can stop the frowning and re-train the muscles. For young people with highly expressive, hyperactive muscles, Botox can stop the excessive muscle activity and thereby smooth wrinkles. This may re-educate the muscles in some patients.[19]

In the world of the *Allure* reader, the fear of aging can only be soothed with the promises of *New Beauty*.[20] With its mission to be "visually stunning, scientifically accurate, ethically balanced," *New Beauty* lulls the reader into believing plastic surgery is a necessary part of any beautiful woman's life. Many if not most of its articles are about cosmetic surgery, and each issue ends with lists of cosmetic surgeons. If you go to the Web site for *New Beauty* magazine, you can upload a photo of yourself to get a "cosmetic enhancement simulator." By using the tools, you can see what you'd look like with a facelift or some wrinkle-smoothing injectables. Then, if you like the results, you can find a "beauty expert" (that is, a cosmetic surgeon) near you.

New Beauty puts cosmetic surgery on the same level as every other beauty and exercise product we are already consuming anyway. Many *New Beauty* articles feature everyday items alongside cosmetic procedures as "options" available to the magazine's readers. Toothpaste is next to teeth-whitening products, which is alongside information on how cosmetic dentistry can change your life. Sunscreens and Botox are featured as similar methods to avoid having sun-damaged skin. A push-up bra is a way of making breasts look bigger—so are implants. These exercises will help tighten your abs—so will liposuction. Even if the articles in *New Beauty* don't themselves induce readers to feel the need for cosmetic procedures, the advertisements take care to direct readers toward plastic as the number one beauty solution. They explain that we need face cream (lots of it—with serious names like "serum" and "formula"), not to mention facial-hair removal (with drugs or lasers), cellulite treatments (with creams or lasers), teeth whitening, spray-on tans, Botox, Juvéderm, and vaginal rejuvenation (so we can "feel feminine again"). There are very few products sold that are not part of the big business of beauty (for instance, out of two hundred ads, there were two for something other than cosmetic procedures, anti-aging creams, or makeup—an expensive watch here, a designer fashion sale there).

O couches its articles in the rhetoric of empowerment; *Allure* induces a state of panic in its readers; and *New Beauty*'s tone and layout calmly assure its readers that beauty is life's most important goal and we can all be beautiful forever. Security will come to those who are beautiful, so, unlike other women's magazines, no need for "fluff" articles on topics like financial investments or careers or even families. A regularly occurring feature in *New Beauty* makes this "beauty is all you need" philosophy explicit. In it, wives of cosmetic surgeons are featured and asked for their "beauty secrets." Here, things like eating well and drinking lots of water and wearing sunscreen are listed alongside facelifts, fillers, and cosmetic dentistry as some of the tricks of women "in the know." Plastic beauty can result in securing a plastic surgeon husband: a fairytale ending for a beautiful princess.

Most important about all of these magazines as cultural scripts is the singularity of their message: cosmetic procedures are inevitable. Joan Kron, an editor at *Allure,* told me that I, too, will get a facelift in a few years. I will have no choice, she said, waving a perfectly manicured hand in the air as if she were talking about death or taxes. "You're too ambitious not to do it. Writing is a young person's game. You know that. You'll do what's necessary to succeed." Kron herself had never considered a facelift until she was sixty-four years old. She'd just started writing for *Allure,* after a stint at the *Wall Street Journal,* and they'd sent her to Los Angeles to do a story on cosmetic surgery. Kron was at a postoperative recovery house and told the photographer who was with her, "Not me, not ever." Six months later she was making appointments with famous Manhattan plastic surgeons and writing a story on getting a facelift for *Allure.* Two facelifts later, Kron published *Lift: Wanting, Fearing, and Having a Face Lift.*[21] Now, at eighty-two, she has had three facelifts and a variety of nonsurgical procedures. As Kron sees it, having a facelift is a way to improve your chances of success in the world. "No one says you shouldn't go to college because you don't want to improve your intelligence. What's the difference between a facelift and college? People know they'll keep their jobs if they make themselves look better. I'll only go so far. I'm not going to be a movie star, but [plastic surgery] has erased some of the stigmata of aging."[22]

Kron is right. Aging marks us as cursed. Our culture so

thoroughly worships youth that no amount of brilliance or hard work will erase the sense that we are doomed by our wrinkles. And cosmetic procedures allow us to escape the curse of aging. It's not that her employers don't know Kron is an octogenarian; it's that Kron's face displays the necessary resistance to aging. But her claim that I have no choice and the claim of her magazine that none of us have a choice must be recognized as propaganda, a part of the plastic ideological complex. It may or may not be true that I will succumb and go under the knife, but nothing, other than death and taxes, is truly inevitable. Still, it is exhausting to resist these plastic scripts.

There are so many rules to being successful. It makes me feel old and tired. I am not alone. A large body of research shows that exposure to "beauty," that is, the idealized forms found in women's magazines, increases our sense of worthlessness and our sense that our peers are worthless too. In other words, show me an ad for lipstick or an article about Botox with an ideal woman, and I won't necessarily go buy the lipstick or the Botox, but I'll feel uglier and probably think you're uglier too.[23] There is nothing to do but flop down on the couch, turn on the TV, and relax.

Sadly, TV can no longer offer us respite from the plastic propaganda of women's magazines. The projects of self-help and plastic beauty have combined to produce a new narrative and visual form: the plastic surgery television show. In the past decade, Hollywood has produced a variety of shows about the everyday pathologies of the female body, pathologies that can only be fixed through the heroic intervention of plastic surgery. Like magazines, these shows are paths of cultural transmission, actual mechanisms that teach us to desire plastic surgery. Although these shows are primarily about the need for women, particularly aging white women, to get plastic surgery, the means by which consumer culture embeds a desire for something else or something more is fairly universal and in one form or another affects all of us.

Plastic Surgery TV

Always Be Repaired
  —Slogan on T-shirt available through the *Dr. 90210* Web site

*Make me beautiful. Make me beautiful. Perfect soul, perfect
mind, perfect face, the perfect lie.*

  —*Nip/Tuck* theme song lyrics

*Television plays a significant role in the domestication of cosmetic
surgery. From the ubiquity of surgically altered celebrities to reality series which make over "ordinary" people, television contributes
to a public imaginary around surgical appearance work.*

  —SUE TAIT

Aired on ABC from 2002 to 2007, *Extreme Makeover* was one of
the first of the plastic surgery TV shows. The show described itself as a "real-life fairytale." Each episode showed people ravaged
by their working-class backgrounds—bad dental care, botched
C-sections, obesity—transformed through a variety of cosmetic
procedures, diet, exercise, new wardrobes, and hair. It also created drama by taking the Cinderella away from her (or his) community and then ending the story with a staged revelation of
the new self to the applause, tears, and cheering of friends and
family members. The show also featured interviews with friends
and family of the participants, in which they discussed the participant's flaws. After one such interview, a sister of a participant felt so distraught about talking on camera about her sister's
"ugliness" that she killed herself. The subsequent lawsuit and
cancellation of the show surprised no one. But by the time *Extreme Makeover* ended in 2007, a variety of other plastic surgery
TV shows had sprung up to teach us that we are ugly and need
professional help.

The *Swan,* which first aired in 2004 on Fox, managed to
combine the transformative promise of *Extreme Makeover* with

the competition of a beauty pageant. Not only were all the contestants changed from "ugly ducklings" into beauty queens, they then competed against one another to be named the most beautiful of all. Despite the perversely brilliant premise of the show, combining transformation with competition, *The Swan* was canceled after just two seasons. Another short-lived plastic surgery TV show was MTV's *I Want a Famous Face*. *I Want a Famous Face* aired twelve episodes about young people who underwent cosmetic surgery to look like their favorite celebrities. Although MTV did not pay for the surgeries, they did film the surgeries and the painful recoveries in rather exacting detail, often showing the patient moaning, bleeding, and cursing after the procedure. Perhaps it was the lack of a fairytale ending that led to the show's demise. Now, however, viewers can go to the MTV Web site and see where the show participants are now and find out just how happy they are, looking like their celebrity idols. Of the seven *I Want a Famous Face* participants featured on the Web site, all of them think the surgeries and other procedures, despite the pain, were worth it.

Two of the most popular of the plastic surgery TV shows are *Dr. 90210* and *Nip/Tuck*. Although one of these shows is "real" and the other "fiction," it's worth reminding ourselves that the line between reality TV and fictional shows is fairly thin. Most reality-based plastic surgery shows use editing and production (music, lighting, camera angles) to create a coherent narrative that always portrays the surgeons as good and even heroic and the patients as happy with the results. The creator and executive producer of the fictional *Nip/Tuck,* Ryan Murphy, says the show gets all of its stories about surgery from "the headlines of newspapers." I cannot say that one show is "real" and the other "fictional" but rather that both are mechanisms by which we learn to desire plastic surgery. Both of these shows teach viewers that the white female body is not naturally perfect, but rather always in need of some outside help.

The reality show *Dr. 90210,* which first aired in 2004 on
E!, follows the lives of a handful of Beverly Hills plastic surgeons and their patients. The doctors are themselves "picture
perfect." Their résumés are "perfect." They went to Harvard and
Mount Sinai for medical school. They have beautiful spouses
and children and homes. They have perfect smiles and perfect
noses. The male doctors are buff, a fact enhanced by loving shots
of their workouts, and sleeveless surgical gear that allows their
bulging biceps to be seen as they perform the arduous labor
of liposuction. The few women who are not patients are either
plastic surgeons or plastic surgeons' spouses, all of whom are
thin enough to be fashion models. The one exception to this
rule is an African American cosmetic dentist, but since the show
seems to be about teaching white women to despise their bodies, her average-sized body does not disrupt the narrative thrust
of the show. The patients in *Dr. 90210* are mostly white women
(in the first season fifteen out of sixteen patients were female
and all were white). The patients are a very average-looking lot.
Indeed, the average size of an American woman is five foot four,
159 pounds, with size 36C breasts. The patients on *Dr. 90210*
tend to be similar to the average American. None of them have
anything recognizably "wrong" with them. While the men
might come in for reconstructive surgery after a car accident,
the women have the rather ordinary problems of small breasts,
sagging stomachs after childbirth, and cellulite.

So why do we bother to tune in to see people who look like
us get "fixed"? *Dr. 90210* convinces its viewers (also primarily
women) to watch it by packaging itself as both "educational"
and "for women." The patients, families, and doctors all talk
about how plastic surgery, like feminism, empowers women. According to the Web site of one of the surgeons, Dr. Robert Rey,
the show seeks to "enhance [patients'] appearance and improve
their self esteem."[24] Dr. Rey describes himself as a "psychiatrist
with a knife." The patients and their families mimic the proto-

feminism of the surgeons. In one episode, a beauty queen's mother says her daughter "needs" breast implants: "She needs this . . . I feel like this will help her become more confident, more capable of going after what she wants in life." Another patient, a middle-aged mother who comes in because she cannot live with her sagging stomach and breasts (a result of three pregnancies), says that her surgeries not only helped her self-esteem, but helped her daughters' self-esteem as well by giving them a mother who is happy with her body. This woman's tummy tuck, boob job, Botox, and laser resurfacing not only empowered the women in her family, but transformed her marriage, re-enchanting it with the magic of romance. The episode ends with her seventeenth wedding anniversary, the whole family enjoying a trip to Napa Valley, the husband sexually charged about his wife's new body, assuring viewers, that "since her surgery [my wife] has just been a joy to be around."

These narratives lure the female viewer in with the promise of empowerment through looking younger, thinner, and more normatively feminine. As Dr. Rey says in one of the episodes, "There's a lot of power in beauty, and by being even more beautiful, it's even more empowering." The empowerment that Dr. Rey promises is about the power that comes from more closely disciplining the female body according to cultural standards. As researchers Sarah Banet-Weiser and Laura Portwood-Stacer argue, shows like *Dr. 90210* use the language of "choice" and "liberation." The women are "choosing" to "liberate" themselves from their bodies by making their bodies more like the dominant norms.[25]

Not only does the show lure many women viewers by promising empowerment through consumption of cosmetic surgery, but it also lures them in by promising an education in what sort of procedures to get. The pseudo-educational format of *Dr. 90210* appeals to middle-class, white women, who have a long history of consuming entertainment primarily in its guise as "educational." Indeed, it was considered "improper" for a lady to go to the theater until the mid-1800s, when clever showmen disguised shows and exhibits as "museums." When P. T. Barnum opened his American Museum in 1842, he also opened the way for ladies to consume without being marked as "dirty" or "low class." Middle-class white women can watch *Dr. 90210* and "learn" about surgery. The surgeries are presented so that the viewer can see bodies from the surgeons' point of view. It sounds something like this: *This is where we need to make the marks for a breast implant. . . . This is why we put the implant below the muscle. . . . This is the difference between a saline implant and a silicone.* Botox must be shot here and here and here but only after we carefully mark it with dots and dashes, a mysterious Morse code that magically freezes time. We are getting an education in what needs to be done to our bodies in order for us to become as beautiful as the doctors and spouses we see on the show.

If *Dr. 90210* appeals to us as "educational," *Nip/Tuck* appeals to us as "just entertainment." *Nip/Tuck* first aired in 2002 and has since been named *TV Guide*'s "coolest show on TV." In the United States, nearly 4 million tune in to watch it every week. It is shown in more than fifty countries. For the first four seasons, *Nip/Tuck* was the number one cable series among eighteen-to-forty-nine-year-olds. *Nip/Tuck's* last episode will air in 2011, marking one hundred episodes, a record for a cable series. The only other show that came close, *Sex and the City,* ended after its ninety-fourth episode.[26]

Show creator Ryan Murphy is openly critical of plastic surgery.[27] "I wanted to do a show that looked really, really glamorous and then underneath you'd see all the rot of everything and just how dark and dastardly and depressing that world is . . . There's a darkness to it. To go into a room and say I wanna change my face that's a lot of self hatred . . ."[28]

The show is not just critical of plastic surgery, but all the usual sources of power—wealth, masculinity, whiteness, hetero-

sexuality, domesticity—are revealed as shams throughout the
episodes. The relationship between *Nip/Tuck's* two main characters, Christian Troy (played by Julian McMahon) and Sean Mc-
Namara (played by Dylan Walsh) structures the show. The two
have run a plastic surgery practice together since they finished
medical school. Although the show sets the two men up as op-
posites, with Sean as the conservative family man and Christian
as sex- and money-obsessed, they are in fact quite similar in that
they are both always failing in their masculinity.

For example, Sean is in an ongoing battle to be a good husband, father, and doctor. Unfortunately, he fails to be sexually attractive to his wife, fails to be someone his son can look up to, and
when he falls in love with another woman, who is both a patient
and dying of cancer, he fails to save her. His failures show up
at work, when he cannot operate because he has tremors due to
emotional stress. His partner, Christian, seems like a success. He
is hypermasculine. In the course of twenty episodes, Christian has
sex with: Sean's mother-in-law, Sean's wife, a mother and daughter team, two sisters, a psychologist who works in the office, a
reporter, a model, a variety of would-be nannies for his unborn
son, the mother of his unborn son whom he meets at a Sexahol-
ics Anonymous meeting, another model, a landscaper, and a porn
star. Not only is Christian successful in bed, but he owns a variety of mechanical phallic symbols, from a speedboat named the
Boatox to a bright-yellow Ferrari. Still, Christian, too, is failing:
his son is not his son, he tries to have a stable relationship, but
eventually tires of his girlfriend and gives her to another plastic
surgeon in exchange for the Ferrari, and he looks at Sean's seemingly normal life with desire for his partner's wife and family.

Real-life plastic surgeon Dr. Robert Rey was so frustrated
by *Nip/Tuck's* negative images of cosmetic surgeons that he was
compelled to create his own show. Dr. Rey wanted *Dr. 90210* to
counteract *Nip/Tuck's* portrayal of plastic surgeons as "scummy
people who are womanizing drug addicts with illegitimate children" with images of "plastic surgeons [as] ordinary people with

families and children and high-pressure jobs."[29] Dr. Rey was right that the surgeons on *Nip/Tuck* are not exactly good guys, but he misses how much the show teaches the same lessons as his own more "realistic" *Dr. 90210*. Despite *Nip/Tuck*'s open ambivalence about plastic surgery, it still leaves white women with the knowledge that their bodies are steeped in ordinary ugliness and waiting to be made beautiful. In the first two seasons of *Nip/Tuck*, sixteen out of twenty episodes feature female patients. Of these, twelve want surgery for ordinary ugliness. These women have small breasts, are not a perfect 10, want liposuction at age seventeen so they can look fourteen, desire an all-over body lift, liposuction of the belly to compete in the job market with younger women, and tried to kill themselves at thirty because no one's life (except for Nelson Mandela's) ever got better as they got older. *Nip/Tuck* is a show about the ordinary ugliness of white heterosexual women. In it, men, people of color, and the sexually non-normative do not need to be made beautiful. That's why Liz, the vaguely Hispanic lesbian surgical nurse, is exempt from the need for cosmetic surgery. It's also why the men who show up for surgery have something extraordinary about their bodies—like a third breast, no hair on any part of their body, or frostbite.

With nowhere to turn for solace from the ordinary decay of ordinary bodies, white women are left with a desire for beauty, which serves as the only ray of light in an otherwise dark and ugly world. Examples from the show of the importance of beauty include: Liz aborting her Down syndrome baby because Christian, the father, would never help take care of a child that isn't beautiful like him; Christian pursuing a woman because she is potentially perfectible—and then trading her for a more beautiful object, a car; Sean believing he can make the world a more beautiful place by fixing what people hate about their bodies; Vanessa Redgrave's character, Erica, getting a facelift despite being a highly successful author and psychologist, because she no longer feels powerful in her aging body.

Far more than *Nip/Tuck*'s melodramatic plot, the surgery scenes instill a desire to cut apart ordinary bodies. Although most of the sets are beautiful—filled with bright, trendy colors and incredibly well-designed furniture—the surgical scenes present a visual feast of special effects that display the body as a mass of bloody clay to be sculpted by the surgeons. Faces, breasts, tummies, and necks are sliced open, reworked, and sewn back up in a way so visually arresting that the scenes could easily be described as surgical pornography. When I asked a research assistant to catalog some of the episodes for me, she had to fast-forward through these scenes, because they were too much to look at. But it is precisely their "too muchness"—too much flesh, too much blood, too much embodiment—that makes them pornographic. To further the sense that we are meant to "get off" on the visuals of the surgical scenes, there is never a word of dialogue spoken during them. Instead, a single musical track, from rock and roll to lounge music to opera, plays in the background. The music sets the mood. And what can the mood be when confronted with such fleshiness, such unbearable evidence of ordinary human bodies and the extraordinary human ability to intervene in flesh and make it better, than one of desire? It is the surgical scenes more than anything else about *Nip/Tuck* that produce in the viewer a certain lust for transformation. Each episode of *Nip/Tuck* begins with the words "Make me beautiful" and each interview begins with the question "Tell me what you don't like about yourself?" The question is not just directed at the character seeking surgery, but at us, the viewer—particularly the viewer who is guilty of ordinary ugliness.

Plastic TV and Plastic Surgery

Are TV shows about plastic surgery the source of our increasing desire to go under the knife? It's certainly difficult to show a cause-and-effect relationship. Does watching violent television make us want to commit violent acts? When asked which, if any, plastic surgery shows they watched, the patients and doctors I've interviewed are most likely to mention *Dr. 90210* and *Nip/Tuck*. In fact, of fourteen potential cosmetic surgery patients whom I asked, "Do you ever watch plastic surgery shows on TV?" ten said they did, with half mentioning *Nip/Tuck* or *Dr. 90210* as shows they watch regularly. The consumers of plastic surgery say the shows give them ideas about the sort of procedures that are available. Of the nineteen plastic surgeons I've asked, none admitted to watching the shows, but all said the shows influenced their patients' desires and expectations for plastic surgery. Several surgeons told me that if one of these shows airs on a Thursday, then Friday morning their offices receive a larger volume of phone calls from potential clients asking questions about cosmetic procedures.

Viewers of the shows often post comments on message boards. Obviously, people who take the time to post on TV-series message boards are not necessarily representative of the entire population of viewers, but they illustrate Americans' general sense that cosmetic surgery is a good thing, possibly even lifesaving. With three times as many positive posts as negative, the *Dr. 90210* message-board posters generally mimicked the narrative of the show: cosmetic surgery empowers women.

> Well I am living proof it works!!! I am a FAN and am turning into a FANATIC! Some people can achieve their looks thanks to good genes, diet [and] exercise and then there are those of us who can't, don't and won't . . . so Lucky for us, there's Plastic Surgery!

> I had tummy tuck, lipo to tummy, love handles, hips, buttocks and chin 4 weeks ago . . . and let me tell you I am loving rocking my new look. I was 15/16 and now I'm rocking a 7/8 I have lost well over 33 pounds and over 10 inches off waist! If you have the money and the need . . . DO IT!! See

Dr. Evans [along with Dr. Rey, one of the featured surgeons
on *Dr. 90210*], life is short and uncertain live like a Rock
Star while you can!

Another poster gushes that cosmetic surgery saved her life.

In my case ... the tummy tuck was my saving grace from a
very unhealthy lifestyle. After I had my daughter I was left
with what is known as the "apron effect" ... sagging skin in
the lower abdominal area that resembles a[n] "apron of
skin." This was very depressing for me personally, and I had
given up. When I did go to the gym I felt very self conscious
of my tummy wobbling around when I was on the treadmill
so, I stopped going. I tried walking in my neighborhood and
had several hecklers yell out "Hey fat —— you need to run
to get results." That was extremely humiliating.

If you have never battled weight or extreme body image
issues, GOD Bless you, if you have, I feel your pain. Plastic
surgery saved me from eating myself into Diabetes and other
health related illnesses associated with being overweight.
I'm now a size 4 and I feel like I have reached my goals.

Thanks to cosmetic surgery and Dr. Evans I finally feel
whole.

Comments on the *Nip/Tuck* message boards tend to be more
about the twists and turns of the show's plotlines and less about
cosmetic surgery per se. Perhaps this is because the show's "fictional" status deemphasizes the subject matter in favor of the
characters. The few posts that do discuss whether cosmetic surgery is good or bad tend to reflect a negative view, as in this post:

NEVER under any circumstances have plastic surgery. Surgeons are not able to separate their personal life from their
professional life, so as soon as they're a little upset about

something, they'll have hand tremors and they will look at your surgery as a metaphor for something going on in their own lives.

So *Nip/Tuck*'s viewers seem less likely to see the show as a primer on what surgery needs to be done, but rather as a general message that there is something seriously wrong with our surface-obsessed culture.

Perhaps *Nip/Tuck* is not embedding a desire in its viewers for cosmetic surgery, but it certainly makes viewers more aware of average white female bodies as "ugly." Cellulite, sagging breasts, flat buttocks, and rounded bellies are the reason the women come in for surgery. It is ordinary ugliness that drives the narrative of the show. As I lay on the couch recovering from knee surgery and watched three seasons of *Nip/Tuck* in a short period of time, I wanted to get cosmetic surgery more than I ever had before or since. It seemed reasonable to fantasize about a postsurgical future in which I looked thirty again and therefore found rewards in work and in love.

My sense that plastic surgery shows have an effect on their viewers was backed up by a study published in July of 2007 in the journal *Plastic and Reconstructive Surgery*.[30] Eighty percent of the patients in the study said TV shows like these had influenced them to seek plastic surgery. And who were these patients? Women, mostly, somewhere around thirty-six years old. They were also primarily white or Latina (33 percent and 38 percent, respectively). They were, in fact, like me (a bit younger perhaps, and a bit more likely to watch plastic surgery TV shows for reasons other than "research"). But the point is that no matter how difficult the question of influence is to decide, no matter how messy the symbiotic relationship between a plastic culture and TV shows that reflect that plasticity, the consumption of these shows instills particular desires—desires to fix our ordinary, ugly selves through cosmetic surgery (as opposed to makeup or fashion or marriage counseling or remodeling our home or whatever else we might have been sold by other sorts of shows).

Trapped in the Cultural Economy of Plastic

The effect of the plastic ideological complex is to make plastic surgery "necessary" in order to achieve the fairytale promise of the American dream—an economically and emotionally secure future. The American Society for Aesthetic Plastic Surgery (ASAPS) tells us that approval for cosmetic surgery is at an all-time high in the United States. According to a February 2007 survey of one thousand Americans age eighteen and up, 62 percent of us are in favor of cosmetic surgery. That's up 8 percent from 2006. Women were 16 percent more likely to consider having cosmetic surgery than men. Young Americans, those between eighteen and twenty-four, are the most likely to approve of cosmetic surgery, but even senior citizens are 11 percent more likely to approve of cosmetic surgery than they were in 2006.[31]

As our lives have become increasingly filled with two-dimensional images of beauty and prestige, we have all learned to try to make our three-dimensional bodies more like photographs—imitations of an imitation—so that we all become reproductions without an original. We can refuse to participate in plastic, but we're still trapped in it. Cultural texts teach us that our bodies are ugly and that the only way to fix that ugliness is through consumption: the right lipstick, the right hair color, the right boob job. A variety of scholars have shown that exposure to advertising featuring ideal human forms tends to make people feel worse about themselves than advertising showing no human images.[32] As a scholar well trained in both postmodernism and feminism, I do not believe that there is a direct relationship between what we desire and the culture around us. A cultural text, like O magazine or Dr. 90210, is read by us, and in that reading is the power to misinterpret. In this sense, the body is a battleground. We the consumers are not dupes of plastic beauty, but warriors in the battle over the meaning of our bodies. Obviously, making the "choice" to have cosmetic surgery happens because we can read the writing on the wall: get cosmetic surgery or crawl under a rock.

But it's not just our bodies that are being fought over; it's our wallets. The cultural scripts pushing plastic, the TV shows, the magazines, the books are telling us to worry about our boobs, not our credit cards. Joan Rivers asks, "Is it better to have a new face getting out of an old car, or an old face getting out of a new car?" The answer, of course, is to take a "lease on the clunker" and get the new face.[33] And how do we know Joan is right? Because we have consumed enough cultural texts to know what is expected of us. I agree with the postmodernists and feminists that we might interpret these texts in perverse ways, we might use them for our own pleasures, but that doesn't mean there is not a conspiracy of capital to make us feel so badly about the ordinary ugliness of our bodies—an ugliness that all bodies will eventually inhabit—that we will buy plastic beauty. And that conspiracy exists all around us, in a myriad of cultural forms. In the next chapter, I will examine how pornography has changed over time, and how that change has also made plastic surgery something to be desired.

CHAPTER 5

The Mirror and the Porn Star
Ideal Forms, Cosmetic Surgery, and Everyday Aesthetics

What a Porn Star Looks Like

Look at these pictures.

— SENATOR JESSE HELMS, urging his fellow senators
to censor the photographs of Robert Mapplethorpe

Close your eyes and imagine a porn star. What does she look like? We all know the answer: thin, and probably white and blond. She has huge, cosmetically enhanced breasts; plumped-up lips; small nose; big eyes; and a hypervisible and completely hairless vagina. According to the wikiHow Web site page on "How to look like a porn star," all that's necessary for this look is a push-up bra, a fake tan, a complete waxing of all pubic hair, French-manicure press-on nails, and a lacy thong.[1] This sort of willful misinformation may be why wiki pages are not considered reliable sources. Even the most casual observer can see that the porn star, like the ideal woman found in magazines, is increasingly made of plastic. No amount of accessorizing can make you look like a porn star; only cosmetic enhancement can make you "porn worthy."

How is it that we know what a porn star looks like? When did the porn star start to be plastic? And what effect does the porn star's plastic look have on our own everyday aesthetic practices? These questions are at the center of the relationship between cosmetic surgery and pornography, although they are very different from the usual questions posed.

Pornography has long been at the center of political and academic debates about freedom of speech, violence against women, censorship, and the role of the state. The questions usually asked about pornography are about its significance in the real world. Is porn bad for women? Is it bad for men? What is porn, anyway, and is it more dangerous than other commercial representations of the body, such as advertising? These questions formed the battleground for what have become known as the sex wars, a series of policy and intellectual skirmishes that were most violently waged in the 1980s. On one side of the sex wars was an odd coalition of conservative politicians and feminist theorists who believed that pornography is harmful to women and children.[2] On the other was an equally odd coalition of civil libertarians, feminist theorists, and S and M aficionados known as sex radicals. Sex radical and author Pat Califia saw the move to censor porn as a "war against the sexual imagination."[3] Or, as porn star Ron Jeremy put it, "You cannot blame porn. When I was young, I used to masturbate to *Gilligan's Island.*[4]

The sex wars didn't exactly end. It's not as if anti-porn feminists won the battle and stopped the widespread dissemination of pornographic images. But the sex radicals didn't actually dominate the public debates about porn either. We Americans continue to have highly ambivalent feelings about porn. Yet in the decades since the sex wars were waged, the very idea that porn might be controlled lost any relationship to reality as the amount of porn exploded in the late 1980s and the consumption of porn moved into the previously unimagined geographies of the home and then, a decade later, cyberspace.

Looking At Porn in Private

The VCR was not invented for sexual purposes, but the VCR only took off as a consumer item when low-cost porn videotapes became available. The resulting demand for machines then lowered their price, making them affordable for everyone.

—MARTY KLEIN

It is not a coincidence that the sex wars erupted during the 1980s. The rise of the conservative movement, a backlash against the sexual mores of the "free love" era, and the start of the AIDS epidemic, made sex dangerous again. But there was another sex bomb that exploded in the 1980s: the use of VCRs in American homes. Although introduced much earlier, VCRs were not widely used in American homes until their prices went down in the late 1980s. It was only in 1988 that a majority of American homes had VCRs.[5] VCRs disrupted the divide between public and private, pornography and home entertainment, and the world of men and the world of women.[6] The VCR brought the consumption of pornography into the traditionally female space of the home. Before VCRs, and later the Internet, pornography was almost exclusively consumed by men (straight and gay in darkened but still very public theaters or through magazines aimed almost exclusively at men). With the widespread use of video pornography and followed by pornography on the Web, large numbers of women began to consume pornography as well. Today, according to Nielsen/NetRatings, women make up about one-third of the audience for pornography.[7]

The American porn industry is a $10 billion industry.[8] Nearly one-fifth of all Internet usage involves pornographic content. The average time spent on an adult site in May 2008 was 5.22 minutes, indicating that Internet consumption of pornography is both everyday and definitely not accidental. According to one estimate, pornographic sites had 71 million unique visitors in April 2005, which compares with 165 million total unique visitors to the Internet that month. In terms of total audience reach, online porn sites are surpassed only by portals, search engines, e-mail, technology and downloads, travel, personal finance, and directories. The vast majority of porn usage appears to occur at home, as well as on college campuses. While porn reaches 43 percent of the overall online universe, it reaches only 35 percent of the at-work universe, but more than half (53 percent) of the college universe.

In June 2008 the market research firm Insight Express conducted an online survey of more than two hundred consumers about their perceived usage of online porn. The majority of the respondents, 67 percent, acknowledged visiting adult Web sites. Not surprisingly, more men (85 percent) than women (50 percent) admitted to watching pornography. Still, let me emphasize here that one-half of women surveyed admitted to using porn online.[9] Since people tend to lie about sex, especially to interviewers, we can assume that this data actually means that more than one-half of all women using the Internet are probably using porn, seeing porn, and being affected by the "look" of porn.

In addition to the porn we consume, we are also all—women, men, and children—increasingly subjected to everyday porn. Everyday porn—the highly sexualized and commercialized images of mostly female bodies that are meant to incite consumption more than desire—saturates American culture. Porn stars appear on T-shirts and in music videos. And celebrities increasingly look like porn stars. Many commentators have called this the "pornification" of popular culture.[10] Porn scholar Linda Williams points out that the process of bringing porn into the public sphere also creates an increasingly persistent desire to repress it. Williams calls this paradoxical "look/don't look" tendency in American culture "in/scenity," a process by which images, body parts, and acts previously marked as obscene—or off the scene—are brought into view and simultaneously censored.[11] Despite efforts by anti-porn activists to stop us from looking, or maybe because of such efforts, we Americans are consuming more and more porn. As Carmine Sarracino and Kevin M. Scott argue in *The Porning of America,* it's not just that porn has become mainstream, but that the mainstream has become porned. The ubiquitous nature of the porn star means that although rarely remarked upon, all of us know what the porn star looks like and therefore what we are *supposed* to look like. In other words, our everyday aesthetics are shaped by the porn star.

In the previous chapter, we saw how the images of ideal beauty we consume in magazines and on TV are increasingly reliant on surgical intervention. In this chapter, I look at how porn displays a variety of images, but the most prestigious porn stars have a "look," and that look is plastic. I consider three types of porn: softcore, hardcore, and a relatively new subgenre known as "porn for women." I am not going to try to define porn, a question that has hardly been settled in our culture. I am interested in porn that defines itself as such and is widely available and highly visible, and is therefore most likely to have an impact on most of us as an ideal type. In this sense, porn is limited to those images of naked and sexualized bodies circulated for profit. There are many other types of porn, such as the highly artistic porn of filmmaker Maria Beatty. There is even porn for a good cause, like Fuck for Forest, an "eco porn" Web site on which alternative-looking types have sex in order to raise money to save the rain forest. Although the aesthetics of these subgenres of porn are powerful, their reach is limited compared to the everyday porn that is increasingly impossible to avoid. Unlike most commentators on porn, I am not going to consider issues of free speech, censorship, the limits of the liberal subject, or even the power of pleasure. What I am interested in is the relationship between pornography and the desire for plastic surgery. In other words, this chapter is not about pornography per se, but about the mirror and the porn star.

The *Playboy* Playmate: The Porn Star as Icon

All societies produce ideal forms: magical shapes of how humans ought to be, or could be, or want to be. The hunter-gatherers of prehistoric Europe had their Venus of Willendorf, her pendulous breasts and swollen belly meant to incite awe and longing for the fertile mother. Orthodox Christians developed iconography to incite not bodily desire, but spiritual longing. The elongated and nearly emaciated images in religious icons are meant to inspire us to leave the flesh behind. The Victorians understood the connection between fleshiness and carnal desires. In the early 1800s Saartje Baartman, the Hottentot Venus, was put on display; her "excessive" fleshiness incited a heady mix of lust, revulsion, and scientific fascination. We moderns have our own sexual icon: the *Playboy* Playmate, a slightly shifting collection of ideal female forms presented to us monthly for over half a century.

Playboy was founded in 1953 by the then twenty-seven-year-old Hugh Hefner. Hefner had the radically modern idea that sex was "just good clean fun," not dirty and shameful. As part of his campaign to make sex wholesome, Hefner decided to showcase the "girl next door." Over the years, *Playboy* has remained remarkably true to Hefner's vision, presenting us with images of women who are childlike from the neck up and whorish from the neck down, but never, ever threatening, scary, dirty, or bad. Something about the erotic innocence of the *Playboy* Playmate set America (or at least a certain sort of American man) on fire. By the end of the 1960s, one-fourth of all American college men were buying his magazine every month.[12] Today, *Playboy* remains the most popular magazine for men, with over 3 million magazines sold a month and editions in more than twenty-one other countries. The Playboy brand more generally, from T-shirts to coffee mugs to TV shows, is up in popularity. For instance, the Playboy reality show *Girls Next Door* headed into its sixth season in 2009. The audience for *Girls Next Door,* which follows the lives of the women who live in the Playboy Mansion, is almost entirely women (78 percent).[13]

Although the Playmate, with her large breasts, flat stomach, and pouty lips, is no longer as relevant as she was fifty years ago when she was one of the few ideal female forms that wasn't fully clothed, the Playmate has played the leading role in creating an idealized form now known as "the porn star." Many researchers have already considered how the Playmate as an ideal form makes us desire certain sorts of bodies—in particular, extremely thin bodies. For instance, one group of researchers demonstrated that although the average weight of women increased in the years between 1950 and 1978, there was a decrease in the average weights of *Playboy* centerfolds, and a trend toward a less curvaceous body. Thus while actual women in the United States got bigger, with an average height of 5'3.7" (162 centimeters) and weight of 152 pounds (69 kilograms), with a body mass index of 26.3 kilograms/meters, the average *Playboy* Playmate, who was already thin, got slightly thinner over time, with a BMI of 18.1.[14] In the first issue of *Playboy,* Marilyn Monroe epitomized the ideal woman, with a voluptuous hourglass figure of 37–23–36, while 2008 *Playboy* Playmate of the Year Jayde Nicole was a more svelte 34–24–35. According to Playboy.com, the average weight of *Playboy* models has increased about a pound since the 1960s, but the average height increased about two inches (that is, they're actually thinner). The average bust size has dropped about an inch, waist size has increased an inch, and hip size has remained about the same.

But if the ideal female form as found in the *Playboy* centerfold is getting less curvaceous and thinner, she is also changing in other ways. The ideal Bunny is increasingly plastic. It is the surgical turn in the ideal form of the porno star that I wish to trace and link to our everyday aesthetics. In order to trace this increasingly plastic Playmate, I randomly chose two *Playboy* centerfolds for each year from 1955 to the present. By mapping these forms over time, one notes some clear changes in the Playmate. These changes primarily occur on the faces, breasts, and the vaginas of the models.

The major change in the face is the plumping of lips. Although all the models, who are generally in their early twenties, have the full lips of youth, starting in the 1990s, the upper lip becomes as plump as the lower, an effect primarily achieved through silicone injections or lip implants. Also, models in the 2000s are more likely to be smiling, and their smiles reveal stunningly white and straight teeth (an effect most likely achieved through cosmetic dentistry).

Breasts are not necessarily bigger, but by the 1990s, the breasts of Playmates are pumped up in a way that is different from earlier models. Earlier models had large breasts that hung down and were primarily bigger below the nipple. There is a fullness of today's Playmate's breasts above and below the nipple that resembles a balloon blown to full capacity instead of the more half-circle shapes of the breasts of earlier Playmates. Also, the breasts of models today, no matter how large, are "perky"— that is, there seems to be no sag at all, unlike earlier models whose breasts often hung several inches onto the rib cage.

While the lips and breasts of Playmates seem pumped up and overblown, the vaginas seem "toned down" even as they are increasingly visible over time. Vaginas are first shown in the magazine in the early 1970s, and they have pubic hair in a regulated triangular patch. The patch diminishes to a smaller strip in the 1980s, to an even thinner strip in the 1990s, and finally to the complete disappearance of pubic hair on the bodies of many of the Playmates in the 2000s. Not only is the vagina increasingly seen and then increasingly hairless, but it is also homogenous in its appearance. All the hairless or nearly hairless vaginas sport a look best described as "neat" and "contained," with a hooded clitoris and labia minora that never stick out from the labia majora. Although many women, especially ones who are young and have not yet given birth, may have this look "naturally," many more would require the services of a cosmetic surgeon in order to possess the pornographic vagina.

In other words, our icon of sexual desirability, the *Playboy* Playmate, is no longer available without cosmetic intervention. Silicone injections, implants, and even vaginal surgery may be required to get "the look." The Playmate has evolved from a rare, but not necessarily surgical, body to one that requires medical intervention to exist.[15] The Playmate has also moved from a form available to adult men to a nearly universal icon of (white) femininity. One of the most popular movies in 2008 among young girls is *House Bunny*. *House Bunny* is the comedic tale of a Playboy Bunny who is thrown out of the mansion, ostensibly for being too old at twenty-seven. The excommunicated Bunny, played by Anna Faris, ends up becoming the den mother for a loser sorority house. She then has to turn ugly duckling girls into hot mama swans to stop the university from kicking them out.[16] In other words, it's a story about how success for women depends on looking like porn stars and success for porn stars depends on looking young forever. *House Bunny* is a perfect fairy tale of why girls should want plastic surgery.

In the world of contemporary porn, *Playboy* has become kids' stuff, the sort of fairy tales you can watch right before you go to sleep with your teddy bear in your arms. *Playboy*'s status as kid culture is why young girls can buy Playboy T-shirts, coffee mugs, and other porn paraphernalia at teen-oriented stores like Hot Topic.[17] In the fifty years of its existence, *Playboy* has gone from the relatively revolutionary position of claiming the sexy images it presented as "just good clean fun," to being so incredibly "clean" as to be for teenagers and even children. In the next section, I move from the softcore "fun" of *Playboy* to the hardcore "fucking" that is so readily available through our computers.

Hardcore Porn: Excess of Desire and Ordinary Bodies

Most Americans look at porn. I certainly do, for both research and less academic reasons. But the sort of hardcore, mainstream porn that is the most easily available can be a bit startling. There is an excess of desire, of screaming (by women), of cum on young, female faces, and even of violence (against young females, sometimes seemingly without their consent or pleasure). But mainstream porn can also be startling for its incredible diversity. It is most certainly not one thing. Unlike an icon of sexuality, like the Bunny, mainstream porn is more like a constantly shifting collage of sexualized forms. Type "most popular porn sites" into Google, and one of the first ones to come up is www.yobt.com. On Yobt, there are 116 subgenres of porn listed on the left of the site, with everything from "Foot Fetish" to "Redhead," "Grannies" to "Pregnant." Older women and pregnant women are not exactly what we imagine when we think of what the porn star looks like. This diversity of form can be misleading, though, because no matter how many subgenres of porn sexualize "normal" bodies, the porn star haunts hardcore porn as that which we most desire.

"Cheap Porn" is the most popular, with 126 sites, but "Hardcore," with 74 sites, isn't far behind. When you click on "Hardcore," all the sites that come up feature girls and women who look like porn stars. They are young, mostly blond, mostly white, always thin, chesty, and hairless. Except for a site called "Black Amateur Blowjobs," all of the images of women under "Hardcore" were white except for one Black woman on the "Freaks of Boobs—Unbelievably Huge Melons" site. Every single image available on the site was of very young women ("barely legal," with the emphasis on "barely"). This was surprisingly true even on the "Hot MILF Club—Sexy Moms Desperately Want to Fuck." MILF is the acronym for Mothers I'd Like to Fuck. If these MILFs are mothers, then they most certainly gave birth while still in high school.

Still, there are many "ordinary-looking" women on the site as well. In fact, the two most popular subgenres after "Cheap" are "Teen" and "Amateur." The "teens" are indeed that, extremely young, all very thin, hairless, white, and seemingly without cosmetic intervention. The "Amateur" site also features a lot of very young white teenage girls. The "Amateur" site contains a MILF site with women who could have become mothers after high school, since they are in their late twenties and even thirties. This is an important and even startling fact: a lot of porn available on the Web features ordinary women, not porn stars. Admittedly, these women tend to be young and thin, have small, hairless vaginas like the Playmate, but they are not obviously enhanced by cosmetic surgery.

Looking at the most popular videos on Raw Tube, one of the most popular porn sites with free videos, there is an excess of heterosexual desire and an excess of youth, but only twenty of the first hundred most popular videos feature the porn star look or any other visible signs of plastic surgery that is meant to make a female body sexier. I'm not looking for nose jobs, but the lips, boobs, and vaginal enhancements of the porn star. Most of the bodies in this genre of porn are extraordinarily ordinary. The most popular videos on Raw Tube in July 2009 can be divided into overlapping categories of erotic desire: teens (20); mothers/wives/pregnant women (19); "large" women, also known as BBWs for Big Beautiful Women, "fatties," and "chubbies," seemingly average-sized to plus-sized (13); older women, also known as "hags" and seemingly between the ages of forty and sixty (10); racialized bodies, usually Black with Latina and Asian being about equal as second-most-popular eroticized racial status (10); anal sex (9); lesbians (8); "shemales" (sometimes called "trannies") (6); and BDSM (bondage, dominance, submission, sadism, masochism; often called "fetish") (5).

These multiple categories of desire indicate that ordinary (female) bodies are certainly available in porn as desirable. Old, young, fat, and thin women all seem to experience an excess of desire that makes them pant for penetration of various sorts. Yet this diversity of bodies can be misleading. There is a definite hierarchy to female objects of desire, and the porn star is at the top of that hierarchy. For instance, in a Raw Tube video entitled "Fucking Mom's Guy," the daughter is told by the boyfriend that he was only dating her mother to get to her. What did he want with an "old woman" when she, the daughter, was willing to be his lover. Also, when you search "porn stars" on the site, the women who come up all look similar to each other and to the ideal Playmate available in *Playboy:* young, cosmetically enhanced lips and breasts, hairless and "contained" vaginas and anuses. In other words, you can be desirable if you're older, fatter, or smaller-breasted than a porn star, but you *cannot* be a porn star.

Perhaps even more important than a hierarchy of bodies in porn is the fact that the objects of desire in easily available hardcore porn are female (or at least "shemale"). The male participant in this porn does not have a look. He can be old or young, fat or thin. Even the male porn star's penis doesn't have a "look." Unlike the images of vaginas in porn, which are nearly all the same vagina, the penis can be big or small, thick or thin, sagging scrotum or tightly tucked, covered in hair or hairless. The "look" of the penis, like the "look" of the male porn star, is rather beside the point, and most certainly does not seem to require cosmetic surgery. The male porn star and amateur porn participant *is* his penis. What plays out with mind-numbing regularity in mainstream porn is that women are desired for the way they look (which can be varied, but always depends on being overcome with a desire for oral, anal, and/or vaginal penetration) whereas men are the penis/person who fulfills the woman's desire. Sometimes his face is not even visible, even though the POV, or point of view, is his. More accurately, the story plays out from the POV of a man gazing at his penis, which is the object of the female porn star's desire. It is the woman's look that is important in mainstream porn, and the look most valued is that of a porn star. This means that mainstream porn, just like the iconic porn of *Playboy,* shapes women's desire to be more plastic in order to be more desirable.

But there is a subgenre of porn that attempts to break the script of porn. In this porn, desire is not narrated from the point of view of the possessor of the penis, but rather from the possessor of the vagina. This subgenre of "porn for women" is worth investigating for the lessons it teaches us about what bodies are desirable.

Porn for Women

When I was fifteen years old, before the wonders of the Internet, a friend and I snuck into the porno section of a local magazine shop and slowly slipped a *Playgirl* off the shelf and turned, ever so carefully, to the centerfold. *Playgirl* was started in 1973, in part as a feminist response to men's magazines, and, although no longer in existence, the magazine was still going strong in 1980. I still remember the *Playgirl* model, lying next to a pool, wearing a big, cheesy moustache, cowboy boots, and nothing else. I cannot remember what his penis looked like, or whether he had hair on his chest, but I remember thinking that there was something incredibly powerful and perhaps even dangerous about this porn for women. Then the clerk came running at us, waving his hands, saying he was going to call the cops on us. My friend and I dropped the magazine and ran for our lives, or at least our reputations. Looking at porn was not something nice, young women did. If only we'd been born twenty years later. Today, you can type "porn for women" into a search engine and watch hundreds of sites, "just for the girls," pop up.

At the Web site For the Girls: Ezine and Erotica for Women, the viewer is told that "women come first" and "we want to see sex where the women actually enjoy themselves. We love sensual kissing slow teasing, expert cunt licking, and fabulous fucking. Be it playful, quiet, or hard and intense, if she's having a good time, we're enjoying it too . . . because good sex is often about more than just getting off."

There is a section on For the Girls called "hardcore" (because "sometimes you just want it quick, hard, and nasty"), but even within the hardcore section, "the guys are good looking, the girls enjoy themselves, and the sexual chemistry is intense." In other words, the women are to have pleasure, and part of that pleasure is about the way the men look. Furthermore, "all the couples photos are chosen because they depict hardcore sex with that added something: kissing, sensuality, a sexy scenario, smiles and passion. These couples actually ENJOY having sex together—you can see it."[18] A similar rhetoric about putting women's pleasure first is evident at Sssh.com, where they "know what truly ignites the female senses . . . Because we are women." On this site, women can get not just sexy photos, films, and stories, but advice on everything from blow jobs to beauty regimes.[19] This rhetoric of female pleasure is radically absent on many of the mainstream hardcore sites. For instance, an entire subgenre of hardcore porn available at sites like DrunkChix.com involves sex with young girls so drunk or even passed out from alcohol that they are not even conscious during the sex acts, which are clearly committed *to* them rather than *with* them.

Although the rhetoric of many of the porn-for-women sites is strikingly different from the mainstream sites where part of the viewer's pleasure seems to lie in the girls' lack of pleasure, much of the visual content is similar. For example, on the more popular porn sites, the actors are mostly white. On For the Girls, of nineteen couples pictured, seventeen are white, one is interracial, and one is Black. All the actors—both men and women—are thin, though the women are thin without obvious musculature while the men are bigger and more visibly muscled. The porn-for-women stars are young, though age plays out differently on these sites than it does on more mainstream sites. On the "for women" sites, the couples seem to be of similar ages and levels of attractiveness. On the mainstream sites, young women are "fucked" by older and far less attractive men. Although the models on the porn-for-women sites are young, they are clearly adults, not the "barely legal" teens on mainstream sites.

The most significant difference is perhaps the fact that on the for-women sites, the male body is meant to be looked at. The men have a "look" in that they are all muscular, hairless, and handsome. Here, men are meant to be objects of female desire; even their penises must have "the look." Under a For the Girls section called "Eye Candy," the viewer is told: "The hard cock. For too long it's been hidden from view, shielded from the eyes of horny women the world over. But no more. We at For the Girls have been bringing you hard cock since 2003 and we'll continue to uphold our solemn duty, happily presenting ever more lovely, thick, hard dicks to female eyes."

As an article on porn for women in the *Ecommerce Journal* noted,

> Women like to watch movies with handsome men they can fantasize about, not run-of-the-mill guys who look like their overweight neighbor. However, adult entertainment lacks hot male porn actors—the performers are typically chosen based on their penis size and ability to ejaculate on demand, not overall good appearance. That's why female-oriented porn movies generally cast better-looking male leads.[20]

One analysis of porn-for-women sites finds that they are a visual hybrid of gay male and straight male porn conventions. "Nude solo shots of male models generally conform to erotic conventions used in gay male porn," since unlike straight male porn, where men are reduced to their penis, in gay male porn and porn for women, a variety of body parts can be eroticized, like the man's buttocks or carefully sculpted abdominal muscles. On the other hand, many of the couples' scenes conform to straight-male-porn visual conventions, such as putting the woman's body at the center of the frame. Still, many mainstream porn visual conventions are virtually absent, such as the "cum shot" on the woman's face, anal sex, and double penetration.[21]

More central to the question at hand—the relationship between porn and plastic surgery—is the issue of bodies. The porn-for-women stars are normatively gendered, young, white, thin bodies, but not bodies that have visibly gone under the knife. There are very few visible breast implants and almost no plumped-up lips. As for vaginas, they are very nearly invisible on these sites—either barely visible under a man's face, or hand, or shot from the woman's point of view and therefore not terribly central to the visual economy of porn for women (unlike the penis).

Like the straight-male hardcore porn, the youthfulness, thinness, and beauty of the women in women's porn might make some female viewers feel the need for medical intervention into their own embodied experiences. There are no older or bigger women on these sites. Although there is no fetish of teenage girls, a relatively short stage in a woman's sexual life, porn for women still limits women's desirability to her twenties and maybe early thirties. Porn for women also creates an idealized male body that may require cosmetic enhancement to achieve. Hair removal, buttock implants, body sculpting, and of course youth-enhancing procedures could all be necessary for men to look like the male porn stars in this genre. Whatever the influence of porn for women on cosmetic surgery might be, it is surely quite small since, like the gay-male porn it imitates, porn for women is a fairly small fish in the big ocean that is mainstream porn.

Porn and Plastic

Lots of women tell me I'm their idol.

— JENNA JAMESON, porn star

Porn is various, but the female porn star is not. We all know what she looks like, because she looks the same. Therefore, by looking closely at the porn star, particularly her mouth, breasts, and vagina, we can see that these particular ideal forms can only be produced with cosmetic surgery. It is impossible to say that plumped-up breasts and lips and toned-down vaginas on *Playboy* Playmates or hardcore porn sites directly implant the desire for cosmetic surgeries in ordinary women. Yet, it is also impossible to ignore the correlation between porn stars and cosmetic surgery trends. Although the economic downturn has meant that there were fewer cosmetic surgery procedures in 2007 (–3 percent), breast implants were up 6 percent. Tummy tucks were up 2 percent during the same time. In 2006, "Mommy Makeover" procedures that include liposuction, tummy tucks, and other procedures to erase any signs of childbirth, were growing at a rate five times higher than the growth of overall cosmetic plastic surgery procedures (2 percent) during the same time period.[22]

In order to have a "picture perfect" vagina, women are increasingly turning to "vaginal rejuvenation." According to the Web site of *Dr. 90210* star Dr. David Matlock, vaginal rejuvenation may be necessary for the "thirty million American women [who] suffer from symptoms of vaginal relaxation . . . that may occur as a result of childbirth, aging or a combination of both."[23] Vaginal rejuvenations—vaginal tightenings and labioplasties, which involves trimming the labia minora so they do not protrude from the labia majora—are increasingly popular according to cosmetic surgeons and the AMA, which officially recommended against them in 2007. Indeed, the American Gynecological Society warns that "vaginal rejuvenation" can cause painful intercourse as well as painful scarring or nerve damage and loss of sensation or hypersensitivity.[24]

Most cosmetic surgeons I've interviewed trace the increasing visibility of the vagina (through porn, but also because of hair removal and the fashion that requires it, like thongs) as the source of anxiety over the vagina's "look." Women I've interviewed spoke of realizing their vagina didn't look like the vaginas they saw in their boyfriend's or husband's pornographic magazines. In fact, one woman I interviewed, a white woman in her thirties in the metro Miami region, told me that she took her husband's pornography magazine into her surgeon's office and pointed at the vagina and said "make mine look like that."[25] The hypervisible vagina of the porn star—with the inner lips tucked up inside and the clitoris nicely hooded—can easily increase the anxiety of everyday women over their own vaginas. Perhaps this is why vagina-specific spas are opening around the country where women can find out what's "wrong" with their vaginas and what exactly can be done to "fix" them. For example, at Phit, "a uniquely feminine" medical spa in New York City, women can choose from a variety of vaginal rejuvenation techniques, from workout regimens for Kegel muscles to labiaplasty and vaginal tightening after getting an initial vaginal fitness evaluation.[26]

The result of the pornification of daily life and the plasticization of the porn star is that women's bodies are no longer in and of themselves objects of desire. As Naomi Wolf put it, "For most of human history, erotic images have been reflections of, or celebrations of, or substitutes for, real naked women. For the first time in human history . . . real naked women are just bad porn."[27]

In order to be desirable, women are increasingly going under the knife—at least some women: aging white women who want to be desired by men. Why sexual desire and plastic got into bed together is difficult to determine. Some hold that it's hardwired into our brain to want the porn star, but I would argue that it goes way beyond human evolution. Our desire for the porn star and her look is the result of history, technology, and culture.

Childishness, Computers, and Cosmetic Surgery

One might argue—many do—that we place too much importance on physical beauty, but the fact is we're hardwired to respond to it. From the time humans started walking around with our body-hair parkas and leafy lingerie, beauty has been an evolutionary tool we called on to assess whether a potential mate was healthy and fertile. To that end, attractiveness is about the survival of the species.

—DR. MEHMET OZ

Beauty, we are told, is hardwired into our brain. This is the "reason" for cosmetic surgery and the multibillion-dollar beauty industry, at least according to analysts as diverse as comedian Joan Rivers and Harvard psychologist Nancy Etcoff. According to a variety of experts, we are evolutionarily predetermined to respond to impossibly circular breasts, small noses, big eyes, plumped lips, and even pale skin. Since we cannot change our hardwired desires for the signifiers of "youth" in women, we must start making things more "fair" by at least looking as if we're young. According to Etcoff, evolution is why we have "the physical fitness cult, plastic surgery, and advances in technology," since even though "(a) man may have no interest in getting a woman pregnant . . . his mate detectors are still firing and he is still inexplicably turned on by a woman who flashes abundant evidence of her fertility. And women are still imitating the appearance of this visually preferred age group, even if they never want to be pregnant at all."[28] Or, as the great philosopher Joan Rivers put it in the title of her 2009 book, *Men Are Stupid . . . And They Like Big Boobs.*

Yet if we are hardwired to respond to the ideal form of the *Playboy* Playmate, why has this form changed so drastically in the past couple of decades? What exactly made her lips and breasts plump up even while her hips and vagina deflated? What exactly made us begin to respond to an ideal form that cannot be found in human nature? How could a desire for unnatural bodies be part of our species' drive for survival? It seems rather more like a recipe for the end to the species, as mates are no longer chosen on genetic traits, but surgical ones.

Despite the science behind claims for an evolutionary need to spend money reshaping certain bodies with surgery, there are far more compelling historical and cultural reasons for today's ideal form. These reasons are partially rooted in our Victorian past and partially tied to our technologically driven future. The appearance of certain childish features on white women, epitomized by the *Playboy* Playmate, is not about fertility, but a holdover from earlier Victorian notions of white women as "innocent" and "childlike." Furthermore, today's technologies allow us to consume more and more of these ideal images on smaller and smaller screens, thus demanding a reshaping of the human body to look good not just in photos and on film, but on computer screens.

The Marriage of the Lady and the Porn Star

Most *Playboy* Playmates are white, blond, and young. Although there are some women of color featured in *Playboy,* they are few and far between. The reason for this is simple: good, clean fun. Hefner set out to make sex "playful" and even "innocent." Because Americans are not so much Puritans as we are Victorians about sex, we believe that white women are sexually innocent, pure of sexual desires, empty vessels awaiting the insertion of someone else's passion. Women of color are eroticized in a variety of ways, but never as "innocent" or "pure." This is particularly true of African American women, who have born the brunt of white femininity's purity, and have nearly always been marked as "dirty."[29] The racially degenerate body was also always sexually degenerate as well. Signs of racial and sexual impurity were almost always located on women's bodies, especially their vaginas: one Victorian gynecologist easily "perceived a distinction between the 'free' clitoris of 'negresses' and the 'imprisonment' of the clitoris of the 'Aryan American woman.'"[30] In this way, the Victorians made white women's vaginas contained and neat, not unlike the porn stars'.

But the true perversity of the Victorians was not that they marked racial and sexual purity on the bodies of women, but that they did so while simultaneously creating the category of "child" as sexually innocent. This conflation of childishness and white femininity (at least middle-class white femininity) meant that we began to desire those white women who could most approximate childish features: big blue eyes; full lips; blond hair. As James Kincaid tells us in *Erotic Innocence,* "I'm not the first to announce that both the child and modern sexuality came into being only about 200 years ago, but it isn't often noted . . . they got mixed together . . . Our Victorian ancestors managed to make their concept of the erotic depend on the child, just as their idea of the child was based on their notions of sexual attraction."[31]

Given the conflation of child and lady and then later lady and porn star, it was historically overdetermined that the porn star would begin to be increasingly childlike as surgeries became available to make her so. Full lips, breasts that stand straight up as if in an extended state of pubescence, and hairless vaginas absent any signs of maturity signify not so much the perfect mate, but the sexualized child or the childlike sex object. Either way, these are culturally specific signifiers that have more to do with the evolution of white femininity than the evolution of the species.

Average Size: Four Inches

Perhaps the perversity of the Victorians can only be matched by the perversity of technology: viewing pornography on computer screens has furthered the need for cosmetically enhanced bodies. Most studies of Internet pornography do not explicitly look at how viewing pornography in the space of a computer screen is different from viewing it as a magazine centerfold, on a TV screen, or even in movie theaters. Instead, most researchers assume that "pornographic images that can be viewed on a computer screen are no different in type or nature from images readily available in erotic magazines or videos."[32] After nearly fifty hours spent looking at porn sites online for this chapter, I have come to the conclusion that this is simply not true. Looking at pornography on a computer requires fundamentally different images than those featured in a magazine centerfold or on a movie screen. The assumption that computer porn can be consumed like other forms of porn seems even more dubious given that there is good evidence that reading on-screen is significantly slower than reading from printed material.[33] The fact is that porn stars who are viewed at a height of about four inches require a different set of attributes to grab our attention.

Given the research about reading on computers, it seems highly likely that the new, surgical porn stars are also the ones most likely to look good in smaller spaces. In other words, Internet porn requires porn stars whose bodies can be "read" more quickly and without as much attention to detail. Cosmetically enhanced breasts that are round, upright, and circular signify much more quickly as "young" and "sexy" than naturally large, but droopier breasts (which could be the breasts of aging bodies). Lips that are super plumped signify youth more quickly than naturally full lips, and bleached white teeth can be read much more quickly than naturally white ones. Perhaps more importantly, the naked vagina, especially in "action," can be seen and understood more quickly as a vagina and not a penis than one that has pubic hair and/or protruding inner labia.

The result of computer pornography, cosmetic surgery, and our Victorian roots is that we desire ideal female forms that are cosmetically enhanced to look sexy on a small screen by looking young, white, and innocent. Having ideal forms that are cosmetically enhanced means that we no longer feel able to imitate what we want. The porn star wouldn't exist without plastic surgery, and plastic surgery thrives because porn embeds the desire, among ordinary women, to look like porn stars.

The relationship between porn, plastic surgery, and everyday aesthetics is nowhere more obvious than on the Web site My Free Implants.[34] At this site, "ordinary" women can use their pornographic photos to get sponsors (presumably male) to pay for their breast implants. "Bucks for Bigger Cups" is one of the site's downloadable banners. A cartoon of a woman on all fours

is displayed under the slogan "Create the Perfect Girl." By selling two-dimensional and pornographic images of themselves—
photos, videos, even webcam "chats"—women can entice men
to help pay for their surgeries. In this way, by behaving like
porn stars, women can earn enough to look like real porn stars.
This ingenious economy of pornography and plastic is but one
of many responses to the need for cosmetic surgery. Watching
the videos of girls who have earned their boob jobs on the site,
one is struck by the "happiness" and "gratitude" they express to
their sponsors for making their "dreams come true."

The "dreams" of the amateur porn stars on My Free Implants
issue from the union of cosmetic surgery, pornography, and technology within the peculiar mix of race and class that permeate
American culture and history. In the dreamscape of our cultural
subconscious, more and more women can look like porn stars
through plastic. Indeed, we can no longer mirror the prestigious
porn star without first going under the knife. And so the mirror
can reflect the porn star back at us, but only after we have seen
our plastic surgeon and possibly taken on huge amounts of debt
in hopes of a better, more beautiful future. What we see in the
mirror and in the porn star is the impossibility of inhabiting
aging white female bodies. We also see the possibility of escape,
of infinite plasticity.

But escape from our bodies is a fantasy, like pornography
itself. Not only are we trapped in aging bodies, but we're also
trapped in a crumbling economy. Most Americans can't fantasize away the truth of debt and diminished earnings. What we
see at sites like My Free Implants is that our plastic bodies must
be paid for—either now or later. The next chapter examines how
the economy of plastic trapped many Americans with no hope of
escape, except through the body. And then what happened once
the plastic money for plastic bodies started to disappear.

CHAPTER 6

Broken Plastic

The Limits of Plastic

One of the myths of plastic is that it is infinitely bendable. It will stretch forever and ever without breaking. But all substances, even plastic, have their breaking point. Scientists recently invented a plastic that will turn red when it is about to break. Such a material will be useful in warning us when a bridge is about to collapse or an airplane needs repairs.[1] Sadly, no warning system has been invented for the American plastic economy, which hit its breaking point sometime in 2007, seemingly with no one paying much attention to the cracks and fissures that had been there all along. Overnight, the United States went from being an economic powerhouse to the source of a worldwide financial meltdown. Everyone in the United States was talking about the Great Recession. By 2009 the official unemployment rate was about 10 percent, double what it had been for the decade preceding it.[2] Some analysts were saying that the real unemployment rate was more than double that and that the American economy was officially in a depression.[3] Whether it was a recession or a depression, everyone seemed to agree that it began with the credit crunch.

"Credit crunch" is a harmless-sounding term, like the name of a chocolate candy, for what was in fact a major economic meltdown that cost millions of people their jobs, their life savings, their homes, and their dreams for a better life. The credit crunch was the result of the deregulation of banking that made paying for plastic surgery with plastic money possible in the first place. When the economic downturn hit, it hit the people with the highest debt-to-income levels hardest. And the people with the most debt were also the poorest. Federal Reserve data indicates that the ratio of credit card debt to income is 50 percent higher for the lowest 40 percent of Americans by income than for the top 40 percent. Seeing that the poorest Americans couldn't actually afford such high levels of debt, the banks started shutting their credit lines down at a rate of 15 percent annually by 2008, about twice what it had been the year before.[4] Suddenly the easy plastic money that paid for the vast majority of plastic surgery in the United States was drying up.

Cosmetic procedures were, for the first time since the deregulation of credit, becoming less popular. Based on data collected by the American Society for Aesthetic Plastic Surgery, cosmetic procedures overall decreased 12 percent in 2008. Members of a similar professional association, the American Society of Plastic Surgeons (ASPS), saw cosmetic surgical procedures drop 9 percent (although nonsurgical procedures like injectables rose 5 percent).[5] This data must be interpreted carefully since it is not representative of all cosmetic procedures, but rather the procedures performed by board-certified plastic surgeons. Many medical professionals practice cosmetic surgery without board certification. Also, many nonsurgical procedures, such as Botox injections, are often performed by aestheticians, not surgeons. Finally, cosmetic tourism is an increasingly popular option for many Americans looking for plastic beauty at bargain-basement prices. Despite its flaws, these data indicate that American plastic reached its breaking point in 2008. It could stretch no farther.

This came as a surprise to many observers. When the Great Recession first started, the stated wisdom among plastic surgeons and editors at women's magazines alike was that nonsurgical procedures would actually go up, a result of "the lipstick effect," so to speak, where people spend on less-expensive luxuries, like Botox, which requires no time off work, rather than bigger investments like facelifts. But as the recession dragged on, even Botox maker Allergan saw sales of its popular facial-rejuvenation product decline by almost 3 percent in the last quarter of 2008. The company reported an even bigger decline of 12 percent for breast implants, losing another $71 million on plastic beauty. Most surgeons in a national survey in 2008 saw a decline in cosmetic business.[6] My own interviews with surgeons in May of 2009, about two years into the recession, showed an extreme decrease in business for many surgeons in the fall of 2008.

The Future Is Still Plastic

Writing in the *Chronicle of Higher Education* in January 2009, I sagely predicted that the credit crunch signaled the end of plastic beauty paid for by plastic money. I said that with 85 percent of cosmetic surgery and nonsurgical procedures paid for with credit and credit drying up, Americans would no longer consume much cosmetic surgery. As a result, we would suddenly become horribly old and ugly, the picture of Dorian Gray come to life on the faces and bodies of ordinary Americans.[7] *I was, of course, wrong.*

I realized this on another run with Allie, the same friend we met in the introduction to this book. This time it was a cold and gray March day in 2009, appropriate weather for the gloomy mood that had settled over the country as the reality of the economic collapse began to sink in. As my friend and I jogged yet again through Brooklyn's Prospect Park, we talked about nothing but the economy. We were both struggling with the effects of the economic collapse. We listed the ways we were poorer and our fears for the future. Her own career, in the advertising industry, was precarious at best. Her income was way down. She was afraid she wouldn't be able to afford summer camp for her kids, a vacation, or even a meal in a restaurant with her (new) partner. And so she did what many Americans would do at this point. She paid $800 to have fillers put into the nasolabial lines on her face.

I stopped running and panted, "Why?"

"I thought maybe if I didn't look so old, so tired, I'd get more clients," she replied.

Americans, like my friend, did not stop consuming plastic beauty. Even as medical credit card companies shut down and credit cards froze the amount of money we could take out, Americans found ways to remain plastic. Even as they lost their jobs or tried to live on much less, Americans bought plastic, but they didn't buy quite as much as before. The truth is, Americans are still buying into plastic beauty, for the same reasons as always: economic and romantic insecurity and a set of cultural texts that tell them "beauty" is the answer. Yes, Americans bought less in 2008 than 2007, but most surgeons I interviewed saw the decline in business reversing sometime toward the end of 2008. The overall trend in the past decade is a spectacular increase of 162 percent.[8] Add in the ten years before that, and we're up to a 457 percent increase.[9]

Internationally, cosmetic surgery rates do not seem to be declining.[10] The international surgeons I interviewed in May of 2009 did not report a decrease in business except for the ones that relied on cosmetic surgery customers from the United States, places like Mexico or the Dominican Republic. A surgeon from the Dominican Republic had seen a 10 percent drop in his business, but that was due to having fewer American patients (who usually make up 80 percent of his practice). "Of course a lot of these American ladies came anyway. They used their income tax rebate. It's been a rough year in the States but somehow they still manage to pay for their surgeries."

A Russian surgeon from a provincial city told me that his business had declined significantly, maybe 20 percent, in 2009 compared to 2008. But two other Moscow-based surgeons said that business was fine. One leaned in and said:

There are two types of people in the world—those who won't spend money during a crisis, and those who won't buy anything big during a crisis, but are more willing to invest in themselves. A lot of people see this crisis as a time when it's necessary to invest in yourself. And it's a better investment than anything else. If your money is in the banks, you lost it. If it's in your body, well, [you're better off].

Surgeons from countries around the world—India, the United Arab Emirates, Switzerland, and Colombia—told me that cosmetic surgery rates are continuing to rise in their countries. In the UK, where the credit crunch has also hit hard, breast implants and tummy tucks were up 30 percent in 2008.[11]

The cosmetic surgery industry, then, is a little like Wall Street salaries: too big to really feel the pain. The cosmetic surgery industry may be seeing a decline in the United States, but in the grand scheme of things, it is still a whole lot more money than it was a decade ago. When an executive compensation package is lowered from $7 million to $6.3 million, the actual difference is fairly negligible. The executive is still rich. Plastic beauty, like executive salaries, is still big, big money. A fact I found out when I went to the 2009 Convention of the American Society for Aesthetic Plastic Surgery held in Las Vegas.

Viva Las Vegas

A plastic surgery convention in Sin City may seem a bit overwrought, like a bad novel with ridiculously predictable twists and turns, but there it is. On a warm spring day in May, I boarded a plane in New York City to travel to what can only be described as the epicenter of American plastic. According to the *Las Vegas Sun* newspaper, the 40 million-plus tourists who visit the city each year and the more than 2 million residents all share the same dream of winning big money. Of course, to win big, you have to take big risks. Gambling is the most optimistic of acts. You risk your money even though you know that most people don't win; most people lose. That's how the gambling industry and neoliberal capitalism work. The vast majority of us are losers, but we keep playing because there's always that one-in-a-million chance that we, too, will hit the jackpot. Maybe we'll be the one to live out the Cinderella happy ending if we just take a risk and finance the bigger boobs, smaller waistline, or the younger face. There's something about Las Vegas that makes the fantasy of winning seem possible. Maybe it's the architecture.

Las Vegas has the sort of fantasy architecture that was first pioneered at the Chicago Exposition in 1893. It is an architecture meant to incite feelings of possibility, escapism, and "fun" in those who walk through it. Anyone who has ever gazed upon the pyramid of the Luxor resort, down the street from the New York, New York resort, with its Statue of Liberty next to the Coney Island Cyclone roller coaster, has felt the giddy sense of endless possibility of the city's fantastic dreamscape. As such, Las Vegas is a physical manifestation of the American dream, but it has turned into the American nightmare.

Unemployment is higher in Vegas than in most parts of the country, and the city leads the country in subprime mortgages—with nearly one in twenty homes in foreclosure by April of 2009.[12] One economist described the Las Vegas economy as "cliff diving." All economic indicators look bad there, but perhaps the most obvious indicator that Americans have lost the ability to dream of the "big jackpot" promised us is that gambling is down nearly 20 percent.[13]

As I made my way from my budget resort to the far more upscale Mandalay Bay, where the cosmetic surgeons were gathering, I was struck not just by the fantasy architecture, but also by the fantastic figures of the Americans who go there. The people milling about in the casinos provide a living map of the American-class body. In my resort, Excalibur, with its daily jousting and Arthurian "all you can eat" feasts, the people were large, markedly large. Because so many of the guests at the Excalibur are confined to motorized chairs due to their size or

the illnesses associated with morbid obesity, a good portion of
the slot machines themselves are "handicapped accessible." As I
moved from the space of garish lights and immobilized Americans desperately looking for a way out by shoving coins into slot
machines to Mandalay Bay's soothing style and design of the
upper classes, I was struck by just how different the inhabitants
looked. Mandalay Bay and the cosmetic surgeons' conference
were filled with the thin, well-groomed, mostly white bodies of
the upper classes.

The only thing that united the tourists at Mandalay Bay and
those at the Excalibur was plastic. In both my resort, among the
immobilized citizens seeking relief from the truth that there is
no escape, and in the plastic surgeons' resort, where stores and
restaurants and gambling were all "restrained" and purposely
not "desperate," people wore the visible signs of plastic surgery:
fake boobs, fake noses, smooth and wrinkle-free faces on the
middle-aged and elderly.

There were differences, of course. In my cheap resort the
boobs were huge and usually evident on the young and not yet
terribly large. The nose jobs and facelifts were fewer. I saw almost none of the unnaturally still faces of regular Botox-users
among the hoi polloi at the Excalibur. In the upscale resort the
breasts were perky, but smaller, the noses smaller yet, the faces
perfectly smooth. Nearly all the bodies at Mandalay Bay were
thin—the result of endless hours at the gym, no doubt, but also
probably a nip and tuck here and there.

As I spent the week interviewing plastic surgeons, industry representatives, reporters, and other experts in the field, it
was clear that these two worlds—the large, plastic bodies of the
working class and the thin plastic bodies of the rich—were all
America and America was now thoroughly plastic. It was also
clear that much of the wealth in the cosmetic surgery industry
was being squeezed from the same people playing the slot machines in their motorized chairs. Like fat from a liposuction.

For the extractors of wealth, the plastic surgeons, business was down, but it wasn't out. More importantly, it was improving from its fall 2008 low. When I asked one cosmetic surgeon why people, especially poor and working-class Americans, weren't just giving up on the project of the perfect body, he said, "You cannot put the plastic genie back in the bottle."

We've been promised perfection or at least a better life. And we still want it. But the usual paths to getting a better life are increasingly blocked. According to a report compiled for the Center for American Progress by American University economist Tom Hertz, the last thirty years have seen increasing downward mobility for more Americans, more income volatility for the middle class, and, by 2003–04, no increase in income even for people who worked longer hours. The only people not subject to downward mobility were at the very top of the food chain (the top 10 percent).

Paradoxically, even as the American dream of hitting the jackpot became less likely, more Americans believed that it was possible. In 1980 fewer than 60 percent of Americans thought that a person can "start out poor, work hard, and get ahead." By 2005, when it was much less possible to get ahead, over 80 percent of the population thought the rags-to-riches story was possible. This was three to four times higher than the number of people in France or Britain who believed working hard could make a poor person rich.[14] But working hard no longer got us very far. The only way out is to take a risk. To gamble. As the economy collapsed, we kept the American dream alive through bodily transformation.

The Cosmetic Credit Crunch

"How's business?" It's down 65 percent, says a woman from St. Louis. Another surgeon from the Midwest tells me his cosmetic practice is down 55 percent. But nearly everyone tells me "it's getting better." A plastic surgeon from Boston who oversees a surgical hospital gave this assessment:

Business was down 23 percent for first quarter. That means October–December of 2008. Now we're seeing some changes though. Implants are going up again.

In general, I'd say that people are looking for lower downtime, for a lower price. They're no longer even thinking about items that may or may not work, such as Thermage. We used to say, "Try it and see how it goes," and people would say sure, but now they only want one thing and they need it to work.

A Las Vegas cosmetic surgeon told me that cosmetic surgery in his practice was also down 25 percent.

Now nonsurgical procedures are more popular because there's no downtime, so they don't have to leave work. Let's face it; in this economy if you take two weeks off, they'll replace you.

Our relationship has changed to patients. Now it's not the same as when money was free. Now it has to count. Whatever we do has to work the first time.

A surgeon from Ohio, who does mostly breasts and tummy tucks, had a similar view:

The economy has definitely had an impact. Started about a year and a half ago. But it bottomed out last fall (2008). It's better now. . . .

I suspect it's in relation to the news media mostly. Telling us things are really bad so we're not spending as much. And last year the companies got really strict with credit—I think a fair number of my patients use it. Especially the younger ones. But I'm isolated from all that. My office manager takes care of all that. Anyway, last year credit got tight, but now it's opened up again.

A surgeon from the New York metropolitan region said that "four years ago people were using home equity loans . . . but now we've seen a huge uptake in CareCredit at twelve to eighteen percent interest. Most apply for it, but few used to use it. Now, with Capital One out of business, they can't finance it in any other way." Another surgeon from a Western state saw the same effect: the tight economy in the fall of 2008 meant more medical credit was being used rather than less. "I was not really into financing until a year a go. Most [of] my patients were cash or credit card, but now about forty percent of my patients are using CareCredit. The truth is, my business is down by fifty percent. I don't have a choice."

Business was definitely down—but not out. Most surgeons in the United States said they'd seen a decrease, but by December 2008 demand for cosmetic procedures was increasing. Several U.S. surgeons told me that their practices had not seen any decrease in cosmetic procedures. A surgeon from Connecticut said: "Look, if your business is Wal-Mart and it's based on quantity, then sure it's hurting. But my business is based on my reputation, on word of mouth. I've actually seen a slight increase in business in 2008." An Alabama surgeon whose all-breast-implant practice was based on volume also saw a slight increase in business by attracting new customers from other parts of the country and even from outside the country. In fact, the weaker the U.S. dollar became, the more he got inquiries from women in Europe and even India.

Looking For a Job? Go Plastic!

It is probably not a huge leap in logic to suggest that increasing economic insecurity is actually driving Americans to get more plastic surgery. Many surgeons told me they'd seen an increase in people coming into their offices *because* they lost their job. One surgeon from a southern state said that: "for the first time I've had patients coming in because they've lost their jobs.

Fifty-year-old women who never thought about getting work done before and now they're losing their jobs, or afraid they're going to, and they're ready to take a second mortgage on their homes to get work done."

A California surgeon said that perhaps his wait list for surgery is a little shorter than it used to be, but the number of people getting nonsurgical procedures is rising every year because they don't have to take any time off work and put themselves at risk of getting let go. Instead, they come in on Monday looking "fresher" and "more energetic." "Who would you keep and who would you let go? Someone who always looks tired with bags under their eyes?" he asked me, scrutinizing the bags under my own eyes. A surgeon from Long Island who has a "concentration of Goldman Sachs types" who lost their jobs said he's seen a lot of them come into his office because they want to be "more competitive in the job market."

A surgeon from Boston with an "upscale clientele" of high-level executives said he was seeing an increase in unemployed patients, but insisted they were coming in "not because they think it's going to get them a new job but because they have time . . . If they have a job, they don't have time to do it." On the other hand, a surgeon from Carson City, Nevada, whose patients are cocktail waitresses or work in the tourism industry, said that with the economic downturn, he's seen a huge increase in the number of patients coming in because they're trying to look better in order to find a job. He estimated that maybe 20 percent of his business is made up of people trying to get a job. No doubt the unemployed "upscale" white-collar workers in Boston were actually just as desperate as the unemployed cocktail waitresses in Carson City. As Barbara Ehrenreich points out in *Bait and Switch: The (Futile) Pursuit of the American Dream,* white-collar workers made up 20 percent of the unemployed before the current economic collapse, but they are told that they have to "think positive" if they want to find a new job. Accord-

ing to the wisdom of "career advisors." If professionals don't put
a positive spin on their unemployment, then no one will hire
them.[15] "Now I have time to get that facelift," sounds a lot more
upbeat than, "I need a job and I'm willing to do anything, even
go under the knife, to get one."[16]

State Regulation of Plastic

*I'm calling on Congress . . . to pass a credit card reform bill
that protects American consumers. . . . We need a durable and
successful flow of credit in our economy, but we can't tolerate
profits that depend upon misleading working families. Those
days are over.*

—PRESIDENT BARACK OBAMA, May 2009

Frankly, they own the place.

—SENATOR DICK DURBIN, describing the influence
the banking industry has on Congress and why real
financial reform is unlikely to happen, April 2009

As the Great Recession showed no signs of ending, at least not
in the places most Americans lived and worked, something unimaginable happened: neoliberalism began to loosen its hold on
many ordinary Americans. Most Americans saw the economic
crisis as a direct result of too little government regulation of the
market. By 2009, more than two-thirds of Americans wanted
more government oversight of the banking industry.[17] On October 25, 2009, tens, maybe even hundreds, of thousands of pro-
testers gathered in Chicago for a "showdown" with the banking
industry. According to George Goehl, one of the organizers of
the "Showdown in Chicago," "the same financial institutions
that drove a record foreclosure crisis, sent our economy into a
deep recession, and needed billions upon billions in taxpayer
bailouts are spending money like never before to defeat financial
reform that would prevent a future meltdown."[18]

As the chickens of neoliberal economic and political policies come home to roost, there has been some effort by the federal government to regulate both plastic surgery and plastic money. The Credit Card Reform Act of 2009 was an attempt to control some of the worst excesses of the credit industry, including medical credit. For instance, credit companies have to notify customers of changes in interest rates and give them the option of closing down their account. Also, credit companies can no longer purposefully try to make money off of late fees by sending customers bills too late in the cycle to pay on time. Despite attempts by the state to assert control, the banking industry has used hundreds of millions of lobbying dollars to convince Congress to weaken key pieces of legislation. What this means is that consumers are still open to predatory lending practices,[19] including the predatory lending practices of medical credit. Those who opposed any sort of federal regulation of the banking industry used the rhetoric of neoliberalism. Republican congressman Tom Price of Georgia spoke out against the creation of a Consumer Financial Protection Agency, saying, "I call this the Restricting the American Dream and Financial Destruction Act." The U.S. Chamber of Commerce spent more than $2 million trying to defeat the creation of a consumer financial protection agency. The chamber even launched a Web site called Stop the CFPA.[20] It warned Americans that a federal consumer financial protection agency would "replace your personal choice with Federal bureaucrats deciding the types of financial products and services that you can choose to own, buy, or sell."[21] But the ideology of "individual choice" rang hollow for over 57 percent of Americans, who wanted increased regulation of banking and credit.[22]

Some states have tried to reassert their role in regulating both plastic surgery and plastic money. In California, actor-turned-governor and neoliberal cheerleader Arnold Schwarzenegger signed the Donda West bill into law in October of 2009. The law, named after the mother of singer Kanye West, who died of heart failure while undergoing cosmetic surgery, requires anyone having plastic surgery to receive a physical examination first. This may seem obvious, but because cosmetic surgery has never been highly regulated by the state, some physicians were operating on patients with preexisting conditions that made cosmetic surgery far more likely to result in death.[23]

North Carolina was the first to try and reregulate the banking industry. Since then a variety of states, including California, have tried to reassert their traditional role in protecting citizens from predatory lending practices. Unfortunately, when it comes to regulating plastic money, there are several decades of federal laws meant to bypass states' rights to regulate banks. And Congress continues to pass laws that preempt states' authority to regulate banking.[24]

The result is a country and a people at a crossroads: continue to allow plastic money to flow freely or step in and control the flow of credit. Banks and corporations like GE that make huge profit from debt are working hard to stop any government regulation of plastic. But populist anger against banks and neoliberal policies of deregulation more generally may just signal an end of plastic money for plastic surgery. Yet stopping the flow of debt for surgery will not, in and of itself, end the consumption of cosmetic surgery. In fact, the only way to really stop Americans from getting more plastic is to shut down all borders, because plastic surgery, like most industry, is now part of the global economy.

Global Plastic

> *MedConsult is offering a wide range of medical services for patients worldwide looking for an arranged healthcare holiday in Thailand. Medical tourism in Thailand is very cheap. You can save more than 70% on surgeries and tourism in Thailand more than any other country.*
>
> — MY SURGERY THAILAND, a Web site for patients who want to save money on cosmetic surgery and have a holiday in Thailand

Neoliberal principles put medicine into the marketplace. They also increasingly dominate how the world does business. Today medical tourism is just one of the many interesting legacies of the neoliberal revolution. The United States broke down trade barriers, encouraged (perhaps even coerced) a variety of countries to adopt similar laissez-faire monetary policies, and stepped back from any attempt at all to regulate the free exchange of goods. One of the goods increasingly exchanged on the global market is plastic surgery. The fact that bodies in search of medical intervention are now exchanged across borders is the obvious result of the marriage of neoliberal economic policies and a culture bent on bodily perfection.[25]

According to Kiernan Flynn, who operates a medical tourism Web site called Navigate Global Health, all medicine is now part of the global economy. To hear Flynn tell it, plastic surgery is like pineapples. In the same way that certain countries produce pineapples more cheaply than others (and thus we buy our pineapples from those countries), medicine too is now determined by who can do what procedures at the lowest cost. All of this started, Flynn told me, because an American man without health insurance needed a $200,000 heart bypass surgery. The patient did some research and found out that a New York University–trained surgeon operating out of a clinic in India could do the operation from start to finish for about $12,000. Medical tourism, according to Flynn and other supporters, "makes it possible to get an operation without going bankrupt."

Although Flynn acknowledges that Americans primarily travel abroad for cosmetic surgery, he argues that all of us will shop globally for all our medical procedures in the future. Flynn even sees a time in the future when U.S. insurance companies will sign up for medical tourism, since "if I'm going out of network for care, what does it matter if I'm going to New York or New Delhi?" And even if somehow the United States creates a national health-care service, medical tourism would still be a growing field, since "this business model was started in the UK and Canada where they have national health systems, but people who couldn't afford a private hospital and didn't want to go to a public one could go somewhere cheaper. That way they could combine, say, knee surgery with a vacation."

Consumers of cosmetic surgery who use the services of a cosmetic surgery travel agency like Flynn's can save several thousand dollars on their procedures. For instance, if they go to Costa Rica for breast implants, they get the surgery, the implants, and ten days of recuperation in a hotel with concierge services all for $4,600 (versus the $7,000–$8,000 that breast implants cost in the United States).[26] Most of the U.S. surgeons I interviewed expressed skepticism about the safety of medical tourism: "What do you do if there are complications? Who are you going to see if you come back to the States and something goes wrong? The implant slips, let's say. I'm not going to touch someone who comes into my office like that."

A couple of U.S. surgeons, however, were already part of cosmetic tourism. Two surgeons from Southern states in the United States told me that they could do breast implants so cheaply that they were attracting patients from all over Europe and even India to their offices. Certainly a lot of their patients were already from northeastern states where breast implants tend to cost quite a bit more. Cosmetic tourism, it seems, is here to stay, regardless of whether surgeons or the government think it's a good idea.

Regardless of whether there is yet another political and economic revolution in the United States, regardless of whether the state decides to step in and regulate plastic money and plastic surgery, none of it will diminish Americans' desire for plastic unless there is also a change in culture. A nation with an economy that is regulated enough to limit access to high-interest debt, but remains situated in a culture that insists we get plastic surgery or "crawl under a rock," is a nation that will just produce other avenues to plastic. Traveling somewhere cheaper for cosmetic surgery is one of them. The appearance of black markets in cosmetic surgery is another.

Pssst! Want Some Lipo, Cheap?

> *Dr. Daniel Serrano . . . was a good-looking doc from Argentina who hooked into Hollywood's social A-list and started giving them what he claimed were miracle injections that worked better than Botox. In fact, Serrano was injecting industrial, low-grade silicone similar to what's used to lubricate auto parts.*
>
> —TMZ celebrity news Web site

According to press reports, black markets in plastic beauty are thriving in the United States. People go to apartments, hotel rooms, even houses in upscale neighborhoods for injectables like silicone for lips or faux Botox.[27] Americans are even going for cheap and illegal surgeries. In Boston, a Brazilian doctor was arrested after a twenty-four-year-old woman died while undergoing rhinoplasty and liposuction in his basement condominium.[28]

Although this tragedy revealed a large network of illegal cosmetic surgery for poor Americans, even Hollywood types were consuming plastic beauty on the cheap. Dr. Jiffy Lube, as Argentinean Daniel Serrano is called, apparently really did inject "auto-mechanic-grade silicone" into a variety of Hollywood's famous faces at "injection parties." One of his more visible victims, Priscilla Presley, is left with a face that one commentator described as "a bulldog bitten by wasps."[29] And across the country and in a variety of income levels, Americans are consuming black-market plastic. The Food and Drug Administration began investigating fake Botox after four people were paralyzed with botulism poisoning in Florida. Since then the FDA has uncovered the use of fake Botox around the country.

A list of some of their successful indictments includes doctors in Montclair, New Jersey, and Albuquerque, New Mexico, and even Boise, Idaho.[30]

The truth is, even if the state finally steps back in and both the banking industry and the cosmetic surgery industry become completely regulated, it will not be enough to stop the flow of plastic. As long as our culture instructs us that plastic surgery is the answer to our insecurities, we will find a way to consume it. As long as the economy increases our economic insecurity, we will be desperate to find a path to a better future. But does the breakdown of the neoliberal economy and an increasing rejection of neoliberal ideology signal breaks in the cultural economy of plastic? The next chapter examines a growing body of plastic resistance.

PART III

The Quest for Perfection

CHAPTER 7

Resistance

Plasticity

In April of 2007, the Chelsea Art Museum had an exhibit called "Dangerous Beauty." Curated by Manon Slome, the show attempted to, in the words of a statement accompanying the exhibit, "investigate and challenge society's ideal of beauty and the designer body created and supported by mass consumerism. Many of the artists . . . raise questions on the human impact of living in the glare of images that, without manipulation, may have no human incarnation."

A piece by the celebrated French performance artist Orlan, who has built her career on documenting her many cosmetic surgeries, hung on one wall. Orlan's *Omnipresence* (1993) is a series of photographic diptychs that document her recovery from her seventh cosmetic surgery. The upper row of photographs shows the bruising and swelling of her postoperative face; the lower row superimposes her face onto Western icons of beauty like Botticelli's Venus and Da Vinci's Mona Lisa. Orlan's project is both a critique of the standards of beauty increasingly imposed on women, especially women in the first world, and a submission to the "need" for women to be beautiful.[1]

In a little room off to the side was an even more disturbing piece of plastic-surgery-inspired art: a stack of soap by Nicola Constantino. In the 2005 work, entitled *Savon de corps,* Constantino used 3 percent of her own body fat obtained from a liposuction procedure to make torso shaped, tan-colored bars of soap. She also constructed an advertisement for the soap using herself as a model. Constantino wanted to underline the fact that when we buy a product, we are actually consuming the image of the person selling it. What Constantino offers with her soap made from her own fat is the opportunity to consume not just her image, but also her actual body.

These pieces of art remind us of what we already know: we are trapped in a culture in which being "beautiful" requires heroic medical intervention. By now, we all know what we're supposed to look like: younger, thinner, whiter, more normatively gendered, and without the visible scars of poverty or childbirth. And yet, even while we are increasingly trapped by our "need" for plastic surgery, we humans can and do respond in unexpected ways. Not everyone is going under the knife to look more "beautiful." Some people are using cosmetic procedures to look like the monsters that cosmetic surgery was supposed to make disappear. These "monsters" are a mirror image of plastic Americans: they are trying to look less normal and less productive and yet they are doing so by utilizing cosmetic surgery as well as the neoliberal rhetoric of "choice." Much can be learned about the world of "normal" Americans by looking at those Americans who embrace not perfection, but monstrosity.

Wholly Plastic

In Katherine Dunn's novel *Geek Love,* the villain is Arturo, the Aquaboy. Arturo, who has no limbs, only "flipper-like" appendages, begins to preach the gospel of monstrosity as the only way to counter the oppressive requirements of the modern body. This gospel, known as Arturism, was born on a hot day at the freak show. Arturo picks out a fat woman, "young but her colorless hair was scraggled up into tight separate curls with so much scalp between them that she looked old and balding," and tells her:

> You feel ugly, don't you? . . . You've tried everything, haven't you? . . . Pills, shots, hypnosis, diets, exercise. Everything. Because you want to be beautiful . . . because you think if

you were beautiful, you would be happy . . . If I had arms and legs . . . like everybody else, do you think I'd be happy? NO! . . . Can you be happy with the movies and the ads and the clothes in the stores? . . . No.

The woman realizes that she can only be happy if she removes herself from human form, from potential perfection. What she really wants to be is a freak, a monster, like Arturo. Soon people around the country realize the only way to be at peace in a culture that demands bodily perfection is to cut their body up into pieces. The followers of Arturism cut off their fingers, their arms, then their legs to reach the highest state of happiness, a state where perfection is no longer possible and therefore self-contentment is.[2]

Writing in 1983, Dunn could not have possibly foreseen the extent to which Americans would succumb to medical intervention in order to become more perfect. Nor could Dunn have known that through the wonders of the Internet and online communities, a new identity would form of people who are not that different from the Arturians. Often known as "amputee wannabes," these people want to go under the knife not to look more perfect, but to look less whole. Amputee wannabes wish to have a healthy limb, usually a leg, removed. Unlike people who get cosmetic surgery to look more "normal" or "beautiful," amputee wannabes are considered mentally ill.

According to current psychological understandings, such persons suffer from body integrity identity disorder (BIID).[3] Research done by Michael First, a psychiatrist at Columbia University, indicates that most people with BIID do not suffer from other mental illnesses and, in fact, other than their desire to change the shape of their bodies, are a relatively psychologically healthy group.[4] In other words, there is nothing fundamentally different about those who desire bigger breasts and those who want to cut off a leg. Both amputee wannabes and women who want bigger breasts are more or less of sound mind and body; and yet their bodies trouble their minds.

A growing number of amputee wannabes are encouraging this sense that wanting to have a limb removed is normal. Many amputee wannabes see their desire to reshape their bodies as innately human. According to Transabled.org, a Web site by and for those with BIID, there have long been persons who, for a variety of reasons (sexual arousal; sense of becoming truly themselves) wish to disable their bodies. Introductory remarks on the site put it this way:

> So you'll ask: *That "thing," transabled, just exactly what is it?* It is hard to define in just a few words . . . but in a nutshell, someone who is transabled "wants" to be disabled.
>
> But it is not so much a *want* as much as a *need.* Our *desire* is more a reflection of the fact that our self-image is that of a paraplegic (or amputee, or blind, or any number of other disabilities) than that of an able bodied man or woman.[5]

Furthermore, the site claims, wishing one's body were handicapped is no different from wanting gender-reassignment surgery. Indeed, the very term "transabled" connects those who wish to change the shape of their body to "transsexuals" who wish to change their sex.

Although psychiatrists are still unsure whether to treat amputee wannabes with antidepressants or amputation, one thing is clear: the desire of amputee wannabes to be less whole is unexpected and firmly plastic. The wish to be disabled is completely outside the increasingly persistent demands to perfect the body that has so consumed American culture since the advent of capitalism.

Amputee wannabes are also outside the demand that our bodies be as "productive" as possible. If our obsession with looking young and strong is a response to an increasingly insecure economy, then what is the desire to disable one's body? If bags under my eyes can make me less employable, it is not difficult to see how not having a leg could make me far less employable. When amputee wannabes claim they can only be whole in bodies that are not, they force us to reconsider what "whole" and "perfect" might mean outside the logic of plastic and productivity.[6]

The "trans-abled" are the fictional Arturians come to life. The belief that they can become normal and beautiful by cutting off limbs stretches the economy and culture of plastic to its breaking point. And yet, the amputee wannabes are—like the rest of us—trapped in a culture that insists happiness can only be obtained through the transformation of the body. People who cut off a leg because their true self is an amputee sound a lot like the plastic surgery patients I interviewed who have facelifts because they "look in the mirror and see an old person, but inside I'm still a kid."

Human Plastic

I used to live in the ocean with the other lobsters until a commercial fisherman hoisted me into his boat and sold me to the circus. Now I jump around with monkeys and frighten children with my big claw-like hands. YAY!
—From freak-show performer Lobster Boy's MySpace page, 2009

Another form of plasticity that stretches our notions of perfection, and also what it means to be human, comes from those who identify as transspecies. Transspecies are people who use a variety of plastic surgery procedures to appear as something other than human. According to psychiatric experts, the desire to transform one's body into an animal shape is a sign of "clinical lycanthropy." Clinical lycanthropy is a psychological illness generally associated with schizophrenia. Lycanthropy is not just a mental illness, but—like amputee wannabes—a source of identity. According to the people who identify as animals or animal/human hybrids, becoming an animal is just another way of expressing one's "true" self. Getting horns implanted in one's head is like getting a nose job or liposuction. Both lipo and horns reshape the outer body to match an inner sense of who one "really" is.

Animal/human hybrids have always been a source of entertainment. A century ago, the likes of P. T. Barnum gave us the "half human, half monkey" or "Lobster Boy." Today many of the most famous human/animal hybrids would rather go the route of the freak show than psychiatric intervention and make a career by displaying themselves. One of the more famous transspeciesists is Erik Sprague, the Lizardman. Sprague had his tongue "surgically bifurcated by an oral surgeon using an argon laser." With his forked tongue, sharpened and widely spaced teeth, a body covered in tattoos meant to resemble scales, and "two sets of Teflon sub dermal implants over each of [his] eyes in order to achieve a horned ridge effect," the Lizardman looks as reptilian as he does human. Sprague has managed to translate his status as Lizardman into a career in the neo-vaudeville and alternative theater scene. Publications from *Time* to *Maxim* to *Screw* have written about Sprague, and he has performed at Coney Island's Side Shows USA and has a daily radio show.[7]

According to Sprague, who has a graduate degree in philosophy, becoming a lizard began as an idea in college when

> I hit upon the idea of using body modification procedures [initially tattooing] for a body based art piece that would explore the idea of what it means to be human from a linguistic standpoint.
>
> I was working with philosophy of language and it occurred to me that some of the principles . . . offered an interesting potential for exploration [by] . . . focusing on how this principle related to the use of terms like "human being," "person," etc. in the sense that people identify others as humans more based on observation of surface physical char-

acteristics and behaviors. I decided to modify those aspects of myself in a manner which would significantly differentiate me from other "human beings."

Sprague has certainly managed to differentiate himself from other human beings, at least in terms of his surface. Thus, besides providing the foundation for his career as a performance artist, Sprague's "lizardness" is an interesting thought experiment in what it means to be human, since we must consider whether he, by no longer looking human, *is* still human.

Another, perhaps less self-conscious transspeciesist is Dennis Avner, known as Cat Man. Avner has dedicated his life to transforming himself into a tiger. Besides the requisite tiger tattoos over his entire body, Mr. Avner has surgically created a more feline appearance by slicing his upper lip in two, flattening his nose, having his ears reshaped into a more feline and pointed shape, and implanting silicone whiskers into his face. More recently, Cat Man has been trying to graft tiger pelts onto his body. According to Avner, "I have a collection of old tiger pelts from the days of hunting. I want these grafted on to me. It will cost another $100,000 but will be worth it . . . When I have the coat of a tiger, I feel I will have reached my goal in life."[8]

Avner has been featured on media around the world as well as shows in the United States such as *Larry King Live.*[9] According to bioethicist Glenn McGee, Avner's obsession with becoming a cat is detrimental to his health and it is therefore unethical for any more plastic surgeons to operate on him.[10] But according to Avner, he is merely doing what his Lakota ancestors did: manifesting his animal spirit on his body.[11]

Perhaps the most photographed animal/human hybrid is Jocelyne Wildenstein, aka Cat Lady or the Bride of Wildenstein. Apparently, in a desperate attempt to keep her billionaire husband, Alec Wildenstein, Jocelyne went to a plastic surgeon and asked him to turn her into Alec's favorite animal, a lion. Cheek implants, a facelift, and some tweaking of her eyes to make them more feline turned Wildenstein into something that was apparently so frightening, other patients ran from the waiting room when they saw her. According to divorce papers, the scheme didn't work, since Alec "couldn't even recognize my own wife up close." So he left her for a younger and fully human woman.[12] Since her transformation into the tabloids' most famous animal/human hybrid, the sixty-plus-year-old Wildenstein has become famous in her own right. Now Wildenstein is Queen of the Hollywood Jungle, dating the likes of fashion designer Lloyd Klein and continuing to add to her more than $2 million in cosmetic surgery with collagen injections to make her lips look not so much feline as like a blow-up sex doll.[13]

Wildenstein underwent plastic surgery for the same reasons many women undergo plastic surgery: to stop her husband from leaving her and to maintain the financial security that the marriage afforded her. It was economic insecurity that drove her to it. Sprague and Avner, like the amputee wannabes, do not describe their surgeries as the result of financial stress, but rather as a search for an outer body that matches the "truth" of the inner self. Financial and romantic insecurity as well as a sense that the self is true and the body is plastic are fairly typical reasons for going under the knife. But the next group of people, who often describe themselves as "gender queers," are purposefully resisting the idea that there is a true self (even as they embrace a plastic body).

Plastic Gender

Gender queers, unlike transsexuals who live as their chosen gender, purposefully blur the binary between male/female in the same way that transspeciesists blur the line between human and animal. In this way, gender queers offer yet another form of plastic resistance. In the summer of 2005, I interviewed fifteen gender queer people in the small New England city in which I was living. These gender queer persons were chosen specifically because they had plastic gender. They were not "transsexuals" nor were they people who felt as if they have a "true" gender and that gender is out of sync with the "reality" of their bodies. Instead, these gender queers imagine their bodies as acts of resistance to the gender binary. All of the people I interviewed had been assigned to the female sex at birth. They were all between the ages of twenty and twenty-eight. All were white, had at least some college education, and had come to this city or stayed there specifically because it is a place known to be "queer friendly."

The city's gender queer friendliness consists of a fairly safe community for gender queers coupled with a handful of medical doctors and psychiatric professionals who refuse the *Diagnostic and Statistical Manual*'s definition of gender plasticity as mental illness. According to the current edition of the *DSM,* a person who resists the assigned gender roles has a mental illness known as gender identity disorder, or GID. Thus, in boys, having gender identity disorder manifests itself as a desire to play with girls and engage in stereotypically feminine games, such as playing "house" or playing with Barbies. In girls, refusing to wear dresses, wanting their hair short, and playing rough games with boys are all signs of gender identity disorder.[14]

Because having plastic gender is considered psychologically pathological, gender queers must usually pretend to be either male or female, but not both. According to prevailing medical and psychiatric protocol, a person must live as the "opposite" gender for two years before gaining access to hormones or plastic surgery procedures and see a psychiatrist during this time. Some of the local medical and psychiatric providers believe such a requirement unnecessarily re-inscribes the gender binary. According to one local doctor, if people do not need to get a psychiatrist's approval before getting breast implants, then they should not have to speak with a psychiatrist before taking testosterone.[15]

The result is that this city, a university town of about fifty thousand, has a fairly large and fairly public trans and gender queer community—somewhere in the hundreds. Again, this number does not include those female-born persons who are living as men. Rather, it refers to those female-born persons who are consciously resisting the gender binary in the material world of bodies and the cultural world of identities.[16] These persons are reshaping their female-sexed bodies by utilizing plastic surgery and plastic credit cards in a way that mirrors what is going on in society as a whole, but like all mirror images, is not quite the same.

Trannyboyz and Gender Queers

Lynn is a twenty-eight-year-old gender queer activist and artist. After taking testosterone for a year, Lynn began to "pass" as a man. He grew a lot of facial and body hair, his voice changed, and the shape of his body shifted to give him leaner hips. Yet being a man was not necessarily Lynn's goal. "I consider myself gender queer. I want to bring people into that world . . . Everyday is a teaching experience." That's why when he used to work the door at a local bar, Lynn would sit with his shirt off. Lynn had top surgery (bilateral mastectomy) and the scars from reducing the size of his breasts and contouring the chest to make it look more male are visible. The scars give Lynn an opportunity to discuss being gender queer. People would ask about them and he would tell him that he is trans and used to have breasts. A few years later, I observed Lynn working at a women's sex toy shop in a different city. Lynn, with his completely masculine appearance, would describe in great detail how a particular toy felt in his vagina. "It's all about bringing people in and giving them access to a totally different world," says Lynn. In this way, he is able to use the technologies of plastic surgery to subvert the goal of plastic surgery: his flat, boyish chest is revealed as "constructed," his vagina becomes public knowledge, and passing as a boy becomes impossible.

Like most Americans, Lynn paid for his plastic surgery on credit.[17] When I asked whether he worried about taking out nearly $8,000 in credit card debt, he shrugged. "What does it matter? I'm a hundred thousand dollars in debt from school. I'll always be in debt. My whole life." When asked whether or not the chest reconstruction helped him identify as a man, Lynn says, "Hell no. I want my cake, I want your cake, and I want to bake another cake. . . . Growing up I identified as bisexual by fifth grade. In college I considered myself a dyke. Now I want it all. I want to get fucked and fuck. I want to be gay and lesbian and straight and trans."

Lynn was influenced in college by a variety of queer theorists and gender queer activists. While attending a local university, Lynn helped organize a talk by Kate Bornstein, known for her accessible books about gender as performance.[18] The moment Bornstein began to speak, Lynn understood that "gender is so not what your genitals are. . . . I identify myself as queer in all contexts. . . . It's more inclusive, more sexual and gender anarchy. I wanna explore the dykey world, the hetero one, and the gay male one." Also, like many trans or gender queer people, Lynn insisted that his gender was not only fluid but ultimately unimportant. "What does it matter how I identify or what genitals I have? . . . I'm a good person and I care about other people. . . . I'm not male or female. . . . Don't use pronouns with me. I challenge you not to use pronouns."

When I asked why, if gender is unimportant, he takes testosterone—which may cause health complications down the road for him—and why he went into debt to have reconstructive chest surgery, Lynn says that he doesn't believe there are long-term health effects to taking testosterone and that, in any case, no reliable studies have been done on the effects on younger female-born bodies of taking testosterone. As for surgery, Lynn says the first time he held his girlfriend in his arms after surgery it was like he could finally feel her against him. His breasts, which were never that large, always felt like they didn't belong to him.

My mom wanted liposuction at the same time. And I said, Why not? The hard part is to distinguish between what I want and what society wants . . . I'm all for giving people lots of options.

It doesn't necessarily sadden me that Asian women make their eyes round or Jewish women get nose jobs or trans people reconstruct their chests. What saddens me is there's no space to talk about it, to question it. We want to bury it . . . But it's not a healthy decision if I or some other person determines it for you. It's healthy for people to have access to choices . . .

Life is art and art is a process. . . . I'm creating a world for myself. . . . Creating my own reality . . . I don't want to be a gay person. Don't identify yourself in one or two words, be the complex person you are. Be ironic, convoluted, hypercritical. But be a good person.

Lynn's words are situated within the rhetoric and economics of neoliberalism. It's all about "choice" and making your own way outside of social constraints. At the same time, Lynn is exhibiting plasticity as well. Although he clearly operates within the plastic economy and culture, he resists the gender binary. Lynn got surgery not to more fully conform to a perfectly gendered body, but to resist inhabiting a perfectly gendered body.[19] In Lynn's world, bodies, genders, and desires are always a performance—verbs rather than nouns. This sense of plasticity was echoed in many of the other interviews I conducted.

Kris, a twenty-two-year-old graduate of the same university, also saw gender, desire, and bodies within a resistant plasticity. "I don't necessarily feel like I . . . wanna box myself in too much. I don't wanna identify as male. I don't wanna identify as a gay male person. Because I'm not. So I'm just kinda wishy-washy about it. Whatever the flavor of the week is . . . I'm somewhere on the trans spectrum but I don't know where."

Like Lynn, Kris decided to have top surgery. According to Kris, top surgery

> really made all the difference in the world in terms of how comfortable I was, and that was a big part of my transition because that was really a concrete, here's the rest of your life as a trans person. . . . 'Cause you don't just have a double-incision chest reconstruction and hide it for the rest of your life. . . . That was a really big commitment. I'm going to be a trans person, not just try this identity out for a while.

Most surgeons, before performing chest reconstructive surgery, require a letter from a psychiatrist as well as evidence that the "patient" has been taking testosterone and living as a man, but Kris managed to convince the surgeon to perform the surgery without Kris's ever having lived "as a man." In fact, not only was Kris not taking testosterone, but he had only begun to identify as trans a few months before the surgery. At the time of our interview, he wasn't sure if he wanted to take testosterone or not, but he was open to the idea because he felt he was "still really perceived as feminine. . . . Let me restate that—I'm perceived as female. . . . I don't mind being seen as feminine because it's just kinda a big fag kinda thing. . . . But as far as people constantly assuming . . . you know, they just think I'm a dyke." Still, despite his opposition to being perceived as female-bodied, Kris retained a certain plasticity about gender: "Pronouns just kinda suck in general, and I'm kinda uncomfortable no matter what anyone uses. . . . With my friends I'm . . . gender-neutral identified. You know, I don't identify as male. I don't care."

Working as a swim instructor, Kris was forced by the manager of the pool to use either the men's or the women's changing room. Kris argued that he should be able to use the unisex handicapped changing room because he is "gender handicapped," but he was forced to choose. Later, after his surgery, Kris enjoyed performing with a gender queer drag group as a drag queen. For a gender queer who has a vagina but mostly performs as male, performing as female onstage is certainly stretching the gender binary to its limits.

Like Lynn, Kris finds that refusing a stable gender identity has made his sexual identity more difficult to name. Although he only slept with biological males before becoming trans, since refusing a stable gender, he finds that desire shifts more now.

> I dunno, I think I'm just kinda here and whoever comes along if it's the right person at the right time. . . . Bodies are at the bottom of the list of what I care about on the whole . . . . Whatever the body is I'll work with it. I think most trans people—because of their gender flexibility—are much more sexually flexible in terms of if it's the right person—not a body—not an identity—it's a person—and that's the end of the line for them and that's a much more queer sentiment.

Lynn and Kris's plasticity—their refusal of the culture of plastic beauty that says female-born bodies must reshape themselves to be both more feminine, younger, and more heterosexually embodied—occurs not outside of our culture and economy, but within it. These gender queers use our debt-driven economy as well as a variety of medical interventions, from hormones to plastic surgery, to shape resistant bodies. These bodies are often coupled with resistant philosophies and politics, such as those of Buzz, a gender queer activist and educator and cofounder of an anarchist bookstore. Buzz, unlike Lynn and Kris, is far more skeptical about taking hormones or getting cosmetic surgery. Buzz recognizes a relationship between capitalism and plastic. "It's all about choices, it's nice to have so many choices, but it's rooted in the history of capitalism . . . Choice is not necessarily freedom." That's why Buzz decided not to take testosterone or reshape his body with cosmetic surgery. For him, he can both bind his breasts and perform as a man publicly and also unbind his breasts and enjoy his fully female body in private. Buzz doesn't trust the "medical industrial complex," nor does he trust the credit industry. Instead, he is trying to live his life outside of the gender binary and outside of neoliberal capitalism.

However successful Buzz might be in escaping American plastic, the rest of us are trapped. We try to resist, but that resistance always occurs in a culture that makes our bodies signify who we "really" are and an economy that sells us what we need to transform our bodies so they match our "true" selves. Ultimately, plastic resistance is best understood by reading the tabloids. Tabloids are the source of much of our desire to live and look like the celebrities (or at least the images of them). The tabloids record our desire to imitate, to be celebrities. They are also, however, a record of our anger and even revulsion when stars fail to look the way they should. That's why tabloids invented the genre known as "worst plastic surgeries ever." Stories and images in this genre are a way of resisting the quest for perfection, a set of morality tales about what can go "wrong" when we don't stop at "good enough." Tabloids, like amputee wannabes, express both our ambivalence about the project of perfection and also the nearly unbearable truth that resistance does not allow us to escape the fundamental notions of American plastic: the body must be reshaped at any cost if we want to find a better life.

Tabloid Plastic

We've all seen the photos: botched boob jobs, liposuctions that leave dimpling all over the stomach, lips that look like they're about to blow open. These images are a warning about the dangers of plastic surgery. In the strange yin and yang of celebrity culture, images of plastic surgeries gone wrong are nearly as ubiquitous as the message that plastic surgery is something we need if we want to be beautiful.

Michael Jackson's nose was done one time too often and the tip fell off. Then, after his death, someone stole the prosthetic nose he wore to cover up the plastic surgery disaster on his face.[20] Michael's sister, Janet, has a huge dent in one of her boobs from a slipped implant. According to Top Socialite's "The 15 Worst Celebrity Plastic Surgeries You Will Ever See," it's "never good when you have a giant dent in your boob. Janet needs to head to an autobody shop pronto, get that dent pounded right out." Vivica Fox has similar dents in her breasts. Victoria Beckham and Tori Spelling both have breast implants that look like inflated beach balls.[21] Tara Reid's lipo was such a mess that she had to have it redone—and it's still such a mess that she has to make sure all the lights are off when she has sex. Reid apparently refers to her surgically deformed body as "my battle scars."[22] And what about poor Star Jones? She nearly died from blood loss during breast implant surgery.[23]

Plastic surgery gone wrong is not limited to tabloids. Many of the more "truthful" men's and women's magazines run stories about plastic surgery disasters. *Maxim* asks: "We heard plastic surgery is supposed to improve your looks. That said, why do these celebs look more horrific after going under the knife?"[24] Why indeed. Perhaps the question is meant to serve as a warning to us all that plastic surgery can lead not to a more normal body, but to a more monstrous one. If that doesn't scare us off pursuing bodily perfection, what will? But it's also a warning about "personal responsibility"—our responsibility to get the right kind of plastic surgery; if things go wrong, which they can and do, it's our fault—not that of a totally unregulated for-profit medical industry.

There's also a corollary moral to the worst plastic surgery ever: if you want to be successful you need to get plastic surgery. It's a risk—a big risk—even for the stars. But, as we Americans have been taught for years, you cannot possibly expect to be beautiful, let alone successful, if you don't take risks. As True

Socialite tells us: *plastic surgery can enhance your image, however, too much surgery can destroy your look.*[25] In other words, it's not that plastic surgery is a bad idea; it's just that bad plastic surgery is a bad idea. According to the narrative available in tabloids, good plastic surgery can transform your life, make you beautiful, and bring you everything you want. Consider the story of Holly Madison, the twenty-nine-year-old girlfriend of octogenarian Hugh Hefner. Madison herself attributes her beauty and her success to plastic surgery. In fact, the *National Enquirer* used the following formula for the Playmate: "plastic surgery = sexcess."

It turns out that popular forms of resistance to American plastic, like more marginal ones, are mired in the same ideologies of body work and happiness, risk and success that the rest of us are stuck in. If you want a better life, you have to make some choices and take some risks. Choose to get breast implants or choose to cut off your leg. But if things go wrong and you end up a monster, it's your fault. You have to take responsibility. The system of surgery for profit is not to be held responsible.

Whether in tabloids or on the stage of freak shows, plastic monsters are all around us. Do plastic monsters offer resistance from American plastic? Or are they merely mirroring the rhetoric of "personal responsibility," "choice," and "freedom" that is at the center of our neoliberal economy and culture? This chapter is supposed to be about "resistance," but perhaps resistance is futile? It's not that these people have escaped our cultural imperatives—they have bent them.

Bending plastic surgery to be outside of "beauty" and "normal" is a sort of plasticity. Plasticity is the ability of a material to bend and reform itself. The term "plasticity" was first used in the context of human behavior by German philosopher Friedrich Nietzsche in 1873, to mean "a force that allows for . . . individual growth . . . to replace what has been lost to effect one's own reformation of fragmented forms."[26] Nietzsche's plasticity is a good way of describing what is going on with the various forms of plastic resistance. It's not exactly an escape from the plastic culture and economy we exist in, but it is a way of bending plastic into forms that stretch our understanding of what it means to be beautiful and even human.

Orlan has plastic surgery to look like Western icons of beauty and calls that surgery art. Gender queer "boyz" reshape their bodies with a variety of technologies not as art, but as life. Women who look "beautiful" and female bodies that work to appear more masculine are all operating within a culture and an economy that sets us free to "choose" body work. Celebrity "worst plastic surgery ever" and celebrity "best plastic surgery ever" are not really escaping the imperative to go under the knife to look good in the two-dimensional spaces we all live in.

Is there a difference between those who merely replicate American plastic and those who subvert it by cutting off a leg or trying to look like an animal or refusing to be a man or a woman? This is perhaps what the French theorist Michel de Certeau would have described as a tactic, a "clever trick of the 'weak' over the 'strong.'" Willfully disobeying everything our culture tells us about trying to look more "beautiful" and more "productive" is a tactic.[27] It is ultimately a tactic of the weak.

Yet Nietzsche is right to point out that there is something that is their "own" about these resistant bodies, something even "authentic" or "true." A perfect, plastic body will bring one more friends and influence than a body that looks like a lizard. But plastic resistance also allows us some breathing room from the endless requirements of bodily perfection. Plastic resistance is a momentary break in the endless quest for perfection. In these momentary breaks one can sense the possibility of an all-out rebellion against the requirements of perfection. What follows are some concluding thoughts about whether there can be any escape from American plastic.

CHAPTER 8

... Is Futile?

Beauty is hardwired.

— NANCY ETCOFF

In the summer of 2007, in a large lecture hall in what used to be East Berlin, I sat among hundreds of plastic surgeons from around the world at a meeting of the International Confederation for Plastic, Reconstructive, and Aesthetic Surgery (IPRAS). Secretary-General Marita Eisenmann-Klein delivered a talk on the future of cosmetic surgery. The surgeons, mostly men, listened as this stylish woman, in a white skirt and high heels, her blond hair pulled behind her still-taut face, made predictions about the future of their field. Dr. Eisenmann-Klein described cosmetic surgery as fulfilling "the divine right of man to look human," quoting the medical doctor William Mayo, founder of the Mayo Clinic. She also summarized a variety of scientific studies that showed that the human brain is hardwired for the "survival of the prettiest." Dr. Eisenmann-Klein mentioned that, worldwide, 87.5 percent of cosmetic surgery patients were female, but the good news is that men in industrialized countries were becoming less satisfied with their bodies. When Eisenmann-Klein finally came to the denouement of her talk and announced, "The ideal body is unlikely to happen in nature," the surgeons responded with thunderous applause. Their industry would continue to grow. Their personal wealth was guaranteed. A plastic future was the inevitable result of biology and history and technology.

Maybe it's because I'm Jewish or maybe it's because I'm just

not that pretty, but the equation of "beauty" with worth, the notion that medical science would cure the ugly among us, and that
all of this was progress, made me squirm. It sounded a lot like
eugenics, and, maybe because this was Berlin, echoed the Nazis'
Final Solution. Some of the surgeons in the room also felt uncomfortable with the idea that "beauty" is on the march and we must
all submit or be crushed; I could see it in their faces. But most
of the surgeons were cheering. There were some whistles, and a
number of those in the audience jumped to their feet. Few in the
room seemed to feel the historical weight of cosmetic surgery's
role in erasing the "ugly" Jewish nose from sight, or "fixing" Japa-
nese eyelids, or "helping" African Americans slip into whiteness.

Dr. Eisenmann-Klein was not making up the "science" of
beauty. There are a variety of scientific experts out there telling us that certain things are "inevitable." Harvard psychologist
Nancy Etcoff's 1999 book *Survival of the Prettiest* reads like a scientific "101 reasons to go under the knife." Among these reasons
are: children who are "ugly" are more likely to be abused; even
infants prefer "beautiful" faces to ugly ones; men are hardwired
to want young (and apparently blond) girls; women are hardwired to try to attract men, and men can only be attracted with
the signifiers of youth; and none of this really changes despite
the fact that humans live in language and culture. According to
Etcoff, what was hardwired into the brains of early humans for
survival continues to structure our notions of beauty far more
than something as trivial as, say, advertising does.

Many of the conclusions in Etcoff's book are shaky at best.
Take the study that shows that even infants prefer beautiful faces,
for example. In this study, conducted by psychologist Judith Lan-
glois, infants were shown slides of faces, male and female, that
had been rated by volunteers for "attractiveness." The babies apparently stared at the pretty faces longer than the not-so-pretty
ones. *Aha!* So we are born knowing what's beautiful. Except we
don't know why these infants stared at these faces. We can't ask

them. Maybe the faces that were rated "beautiful" were simply the faces that looked "good" (more symmetrical) in two-dimensional space? That would certainly fit with much of what we know of cosmetic surgery and its relationship to advertising and film stars. Some faces that look great onstage don't play the same on film or in print. Maybe what these babies could see in the "pretty" faces were clearly defined features that were easily recognizable? Ultimately there is a difference in looking at a real face and the representation of one in a photograph. Surely we are not hardwired to prefer two dimensions over three?

A few pages later in Etcoff's book, we learn that a disproportionate number of abused children are ugly. This study was based on children in the court system, thus these children were more likely to be from poor and uneducated families because those are the children most likely to end up in court protection (if not the most likely to be abused). It could be that poverty leaves its marks on children—bad haircuts, bad dental care, unhealthy diets. It could also be that poor kids just don't look "cute" to whoever is rating them as unattractive (in this case, no doubt university students working as research assistants).

But let's just say it's true and we are more likely to abuse children who are not pretty. What could that prove about evolution? We're not cavemen. We're consumers trapped in a culture that demands that we be beautiful. If we don't like our ugly kids as much as the cute kids on TV, is that proof of being hardwired for beauty or socialized to believe that beauty is good and ugly is bad?[1]

In addition to Dr. Etcoff, a variety of other experts are willing to tell us that being "ugly" is no longer an option if you want to be part of the gene pool. In *The Power and Paradox of Physical Attractiveness,* Gordon Patzer makes a claim similar to Etcoff's about the universal nature of beauty. "Physical attractiveness . . . transcends time, geography, and culture."[2] In *Looks: Why They Matter More Than You Ever Imagined,* Dr. Patzer marshals the evidence to show that if beauty attracts, a healthy, youthful appearance is attractive because it signifies reproductive capability. Men are attracted to younger women because their youth signifies this potential. Women's attraction to slightly older men rests on the assumption that an older man may have more resources to offer her children, enhancing the possibility that they will survive long enough to reproduce themselves.[3]

Sure, this sort of "evolutionary biology" ignores culture and economy.[4] Sure, it ignores much of the evolutionary record as well (humans did not always live in dyadic couplings, à la Man big hunter, Woman stay in cave and raise children). And yet, this is the sort of scientific evidence that we are bombarded with. This sort of science makes it seem like we have no choice but to pursue eternal youth for women and strength for men.

But it's not just the scientists making these claims; journalists often translate the results of bad science into easily digested sound bites that are even worse than the original findings. Take the case of a study in which women were said to show a preference for attractive babies. The study, based on small numbers and drawing broad conclusions, was conducted by two of Etcoff's colleagues at McLean Hospital, Rinah Yamamoto and Igor Elman, and utilized twenty-seven volunteers, thirteen women and fourteen men. When the subjects were shown photos of "beautiful" and "ugly" babies on a computer screen, the women were more likely to turn away from the "ugly" images more quickly than the "beautiful" ones. The study concludes that the female subjects' unwillingness to look at "ugly" babies—who had a cleft palate, Down syndrome, or fetal alcohol syndrome—may reflect an "evolutionary-derived need for diversion of limited resources to the nurturance of healthy offspring."[5]

It is a big leap to go from thirteen women who were probably students at Harvard Medical School to all women at all times. But let's say all women are likely to turn away from these photos. How do we know it's evolution and not twenty-first-century American visual culture driving this response? Wouldn't we need to compare these women with women existing outside late consumer capitalism to make this determination? Is it not possible that the women were just feeling sad that the babies were born with disabilities? What if the women were feeling empathy rather than disgust? But never mind these questions, because the media was happy to announce, based on these findings, that "moms hate ugly offspring." As Jeffrey Kluger wrote in *Time* magazine: "Turns out that your mother's feelings for you may not be the unconditional things you always assumed. It's possible, researchers say, that the prettier you were when you were born, the more she loved you."[6] *Amateur Scientist* read the study this way: "Women hate ugly babies . . . proving once and for all that the expression 'a face only a mother could love' is utterly meaningless."[7]

And it's not just journalists covering bad science feeding the flames of our beauty obsession. It's everywhere you look: there is that single, unobtainable standard of beauty that makes cosmetic surgery inevitable. Even that perfect symbol of the American psyche, Homer Simpson, teaches us to want cosmetic surgery. In an episode titled "Husbands and Knives," Homer realizes that he can no longer keep up with his newly successful wife, Marge. So Homer gets a variety of surgeries—including stomach stapling, liposuction, a full body lift, and hair plugs. At the end of the episode, when Homer is returned to his regular Everyman form, his daughter Lisa says, "I hope you've learned something." Homer responds, "I sure have. Plastic surgery is a mistake because it hasn't been perfected yet to where you look really good. When it is, everyone should get it!" To which Bart responds, "Amen!"[8]

Everyone's Going Plastic. Even Me?

Buy a copy of this book so Laurie Essig can have the facelift she wants and is trying to talk herself out of.
—*Allure* editor Joan Kron's suggested blurb for *American Plastic*

It certainly seems like everyone is getting cosmetic surgery, or will eventually. A recent beauty pageant in Budapest, Miss Plastic Hungary 2009, was not just a competition between women, but a competition among the plastic surgeons who had sculpted the contestants.[9] Even beauty queens have to "improve" their look. At one plastic surgery conference, I was introduced to a company called Beauty for Life, which promotes cosmetic surgery across the life span, beginning with teenagers. According to the company's Web site,

> Plastic surgery can shape the nose, reset the ears, and balance the chest, so that teens can focus on school, sports, socializing, and fun . . . These procedures help boost confidence during these critical years of development.
>
> Combined with good teen health—based on a balanced diet, lots of exercise, using sunscreen, and avoiding smoking—cosmetic procedures help many teens feel more comfortable and confident in their own skin.[10]

So now raising healthy teenagers involves encouraging them to get cosmetic work done—whether it be breast augmentation or laser skin resurfacing.

In my field notes I wrote: *And what's next? Cosmetic surgery for babies?* If the beauty scientists are right and ugly children aren't treated as well as beautiful children, and ugly adults don't earn as much money or achieve as much success, then don't we owe it to our children to give them every chance possible by getting their physical appearance fixed? And is it too far-fetched to imagine a time when no child will be born ugly? When we are able to alter babies in utero so that they never have to face a day as an unattractive person?

I'm not above all this. My children happen to be beautiful and "normal," and if we are to believe writers like Etcoff and Patzer, that's why I love them so much. But what if my children were unattractive and wanted to "fix" something? Would I stop them? I might encourage them to look at all the facts, the risks, the results, the financial costs, as well as the opportunity costs of getting work done. But I rather doubt that if one of my children came to me and said, "I'm too depressed to go to school" because of x, y, or z that I'd respond with, "You'll just have to live with it" or "It's what's on the inside that counts." Good parenting won't change the fact that if you're "ugly," you'll have fewer opportunities than if you're "beautiful."

Contemporary middle-class parenting is all about providing "opportunities." I create opportunities for my children to eat healthily and exercise regularly. Of course, that's different than providing surgical opportunities, it's about health, but it's also about hoping that by looking and acting middle class, my children will manage to stay in the middle class, something that is far from guaranteed given the past thirty years of downward economic mobility for most Americans. Encouraging the bodily habits of the middle class is not that different from making my children do their homework and encouraging them to do well in school. I'm worried about their futures; so are the parents who take out a loan so their sixteen-year-old daughter can get breast implants.

A lot of us are scared. And sometimes beauty seems like the only way to stay afloat in a country where it's every man, woman, and child for themselves. I too grab onto beauty in hopes it will help me survive. I am most certainly not against beauty. I am not even against commercial beauty. I dye my hair, wax, shave, work out, and spend an inordinate amount of time on what to wear. I tell myself that my beauty habits are healthy or at least not unhealthy. I use organic and cruelty-free cosmetics and hair dye. I try to buy clothes that weren't made in sweatshops. I try to work out for strength rather than thinness. But who am I kidding? I'm as insecure (and vain) as the next person, and the amount of money I spend on my "wild-mushroom-derived" anti-wrinkle cream can only be described as obscene.

People often point this out to me during my talks. As if my own beauty habits mean that I cannot critique the plastic ideological and industrial complex and the debt that drives it. They say: "Gee, nice haircut. And where did you get those fabulous boots? And doesn't looking good undermine your point?" But I refuse to believe that our only choices are either to give up completely on looking "good" or to submit to heroic medical intervention. The culture may tell us we have no choice but to go under the knife, and banks may be there to pave the way with high-interest loans, but we actually do not have to pay thousands of dollars and risk our lives to look "good."

Homer Simpson Is Wrong

Mass Production for Volvos, not Vulvas!

Long Live Long Labia!
   —Signs at a street rally protesting cosmetic vaginal surgery

Enough is as good as a feast.
                                    —MARY POPPINS

I'm going to go out on a limb here and say that Homer Simpson is wrong. We have some choices to make. We can actually express some agency. We can even resist. We can change our definition of what looks "good." If human history shows us that beauty is hardwired into our brains, it also shows us that culture defines what beauty is. Even a cursory look at other times and places shows us that. If you don't believe me, pick up a *Na-*

tional Geographic or a history of fashion. Or just look around you. Isn't "urban" beauty different from "rural"? Or what's beautiful to teenagers versus fifty-year-olds? And how about class differences in beauty? Are sexually desirable working-class men really the same as rich studs? And what about national differences in beauty? Aren't French beauties different from Americans ones? And what about sexual identities? Aren't gay bars crowded with people who look different from those who go to straight bars? Whatever beauty is, it is most certainly not one thing. We must resist scientific and popular culture claims that beauty is universal and that we should all strive to look the same.

We must create institutional structures to regulate banking and medicine. In the UK and France there are calls for increased regulation of not just cosmetic surgery, but any and all advertising for aesthetic surgery.[11]

In addition to regulation, we can reward those companies that are themselves not selling us a "universal" and unobtainable standard of beauty. The Dove "Real Beauty" campaign is a good example of what corporations can do differently. By using women of various shapes and sizes, by creating ads that show consumers how makeup, lighting, and airbrushing turn beautiful models into "perfect" ones, Dove is helping to dismantle the claim that the beautiful body can no longer be found in nature. The Dove ads feature a variety of female forms looking both beautiful and far from perfect. When the Dove soap company started its "Real Beauty" campaign in 2004, about three-quarters of women wanted more realistic images of women used in advertising. In 2009 nearly 100 percent of women surveyed wanted women in advertisements to be real, not airbrushed, and for ads to feature models of different shapes and sizes.[12] Like all corporations, Dove is trying to sell us something for a profit. And no, none of us need soaps and creams. But if we are going to buy them, and at this point most of us are, then at least there are companies that are selling products without selling insecurity by featuring "perfect" models (whose perfection is inevitably achieved via airbrushing and/or surgical enhancement).

Above all, we need to create alternative cultures of beauty that do not require surgery or debt. And culture is not an individual project. We must work with other people to create it. One such attempt to create an alternative to commercial beauty culture is the International Vulva Knitting Circle, which formed to resist social pressures for vaginal cosmetic surgery.[13] According to the group's founders, in promoting and performing vaginal aesthetic surgery, cosmetic surgeons are playing on deep-seated cultural disgust and shame associated with the vagina.[14] Two of the group's members, Rachel Liebert and Tash Wong, point out that vaginas are hidden in our culture. Unlike breasts or faces, vaginas aren't visible as we're walking down the street. We don't look at them in the locker room. Everything we know about them is from porn, or advertising telling us there's something wrong "down there." The knitting circle sought to counter that by inviting people, mostly women, to engage in the ordinary activity of knitting while also talking about vaginas. According to Liebert, "It's our bodies and everyday of our life we can get up and decide to do things or not to do things. We can get up and talk to each other."[15]

Of course, few of us are going to join a vulva knitting circle—if for no other reason than that few of us know how to knit. But there are other ways to recognize that we do not have to respond like Pavlov's dogs every time a surgeon tries to tell us there's something wrong with our bodies and the problem must be fixed. We can form "reality check" groups to critique our relentless pursuit of perfect beauty at any cost. I'm going to start one immediately. I'm turning forty-five this year and, like most Americans, my job is far from secure. I think if I looked younger and less "tired," then I'd be more likely to keep my job or get a new one. Spending $5,000 on cosmetic procedures

would involve not going on vacation with my children and ...
being able to buy any clothes this year, but the truth is, I would
be more "marketable" if I did. I secretly hope my reality-check
group will tell me not to do it—that the fight against aging is a
losing battle and it's throwing good money after a bad idea. But
if they approve, then I'm pretty sure a mid-facelift and some
fillers are in order.

If you come to your reality-check group with the desire for
a facelift, and after discussing the financial and health risks involved, you decide to do it anyway, then you will at least be
making a far more informed and realistic choice than if you sit
at home alone and watch plastic surgery shows while you try to
pay your bills and fantasize that if only you looked better you'd
have more money because your career would suddenly take off
or Prince Charming would finally show up, haul you up onto the
back of his horse, and ride off with you. Reality-check groups
could help young women weigh thousands of dollars in high-
interest debt for cosmetic surgery against opportunity costs:
education, travel, or just paying the rent. Having boobs like
Pamela Anderson is not going to make you "the sexiest woman
alive." Having a nose job like Ashley Tisdale's is not going to
make you a Disney star.

We can also read culture critically rather than accepting "com-
monsense" ideas as true: "Ah, this ad is telling me that Botox is
about 'freedom of expression,' but Botox is actually a product that
paralyzes human expression. How cynical of them. I'm not buying it." Or, "Gee, why do all the American newscasters look so
different from, say, the British ones? Oh, they've had some work
done?" Or, "The porn star is not a real person and can only exist
as a product of surgery."

We must demand economic reform too. We can parlay our
reality-check groups into something bigger. Rather than being satisfied with the individual project of "making it," we can

think about the structural conditions that make us so insecure in the first place. And do something about them. We must work together to get the cosmetic surgery industry regulated. But we also have to stop ignoring the money and the power behind all this. No more unregulated banking. No more debt for dreams of a better future—whether it's a subprime mortgage, a high-interest student loan, or a boob job on a credit card. We must demand fundamental economic and political reform. We can no longer bury our heads in the sand, or the pile of beauty magazines we store in our bathrooms. The economy and state are not separate from what we see in the mirror.

We can also be realistic about our own futures. Getting a face-lift or boob job is not going to change the structure of our economy and society. We cannot solve downward mobility for most Americans, unequal pay for women for the same work, or lack of opportunity for poor and working-class Americans through individual forms of consumption. Structural problems require structural solutions. Boob jobs and lipo are not going to bring about economic and social justice.

We must join together in our reality-check groups to counter the dementia of American plastic and the American dream. We cannot keep consuming more and more on plastic money. We cannot spend all our time and resources on the impossible project of perfection, especially the perfect body. With two wars still eating up most of the country's resources, an economic collapse, and an environmental disaster of unimaginable proportions, it's time to introduce some reality into the American dream. We cannot continue to dream of our own future success even as most of us are getting worse off. "Making it" is not only less likely as income shifts to the richest—it's also less ethical. We have to change "making it" to mean making it in a world where everyone has access to opportunities, including the opportunity for a good education without debt, as well as more basic needs like shelter, food, and healthcare.

In *Bright-Sided: How the Relentless Promotion of Positive Thinking Has Undermined America,* Barbara Ehrenreich also offers reality as an alternative to the American dream. Ehrenreich suggests that, rather than insisting on the positive thinking of "I'm gonna make it someday if I just . . ." or the negative thinking of depression, we actually "try to get outside of ourselves and see things 'as they are,' or as uncolored as possible by our own feelings and fantasies to understand that the world is full of both danger and opportunity—the chance of great happiness as well as the certainty of death."[16]

But we Americans are so divorced from reality that we no longer even believe death is guaranteed. Inventor and technology guru Ray Kurzweil has been predicting the near immortality of humans, or at least human/computer hybrids, for over a decade. And he's not insane. He's just more up on technologies, especially robotics and nanotechnologies, than the rest of us. According to Kurzweil, if you're under thirty, you will live as long as you want to.[17] But as Bill Jay, computer geek extraordinaire, points out in his essay "Why the Future Doesn't Need Us," just because the technology might exist, does not mean we have to pursue it.[18]

We don't have to live forever and we don't have to look young forever. That is not the same as giving up on "beauty." Most research shows that humans create reality through interaction with their peers. We compare ourselves with our peers; we get our sense of what sociologist Erving Goffman called "the definition of the situation" from the people we hang out with.[19] But if your peers are mere projections on the TV or computer screen, that's bad for your sense of reality. Sit around with other actual humans. Knit vulvas or make the decision to get a designer vulva. But think it through with actual humans and actual facts and figures about what things really cost and what the future might actually hold. Then, and only then, can we reinvent ourselves and our country—not as a perfect dreamscape of endless opportunity, but a place where opportunity is evenly distributed throughout the population and our lives are not perfect, but good enough. Only when we stop seeking perfection, and rather demand a society that is good enough for everyone, can America become not plastic but real.

Acknowledgments

A book is always a group project, the result of individuals as well as institutions. This book is no exception. I want to thank my editor, Gayatri Patnaik, and my first agent, Anna Ghosh, for believing in this book and in me. I owe my employer, Middlebury College, my gratitude for institutional support in the form of research funds, money for conferences, and providing me with research assistants. I especially want to thank Jim Ralph, who made that institutional support happen. Sociology/Anthropology and Women and Gender Studies provided me with enough collegial support and space to pursue this work. I am also indebted to my other institutional homes—the Chellis House, the Queer Studies House, and the Center for the Comparative Study of Race and Ethnicity—for their support and for inviting me to present this work in various stages.

Middlebury College also provides me with some of the best colleagues and students in the world. In particular, I'd like to thank Roman Graf, Sujata Moorti, Kevin Moss, Ellen Oxfeld, Peggy Nelson, and William Poulin-Deltour for listening to me blather on about this book and never once telling me to shut up. My comrades Linus van Pelt and Rebecca Tiger questioned my ideas, read drafts, and generally entertained me with many hours of fun. I'd also like to thank the many students who helped me with this project, including my research assistants Tamara Vatnick, Molli Freeman-Lynde, and especially Christine Bachman for her heroic work as first reader of this manuscript.

Friends at other institutions also provided insights, ideas, and interest, including Beth Mintz and Moustapha Diouf at the University of Vermont, David Napier at University College

London, Robert Vanderbeck at Leeds University, and Shirley Collado at Lafayette. I especially want to thank Costas Lapavitsas, at University of London, for his endless explanations of all things economic. And then there are my super-smart and super-excellent writer friends who are always willing to talk to me about this or any other project, especially Judith Levine and my cousin Todd Essig, who not only writes but has a day job as a psychologist.

Finally, I owe an inordinate debt to the many consumers of cosmetic surgery and cosmetic surgeons who took the time to speak with me. I especially want to thank Chris McEwan and Joan Kron for their time and insight. In addition, to the wonderful people at the International Confederation for Plastic, Reconstructive, and Aesthetic Surgery (IPRAS) and the American Society for Aesthetic Plastic Surgery (ASAPS), as well as the people at Cosmetic Surgery EXPO for letting me crash their conferences and pretend to be "press," thank you. And speaking of "press," thank you to my editors at *True/Slant,* especially Coates Bateman, for letting me write endlessly about American plastic and anything else that caught my eye.

Books don't happen just at work; they happen at home too. I am eternally indebted to Ximena Mejia, for showing up at the end of this project, just in time to make my life far less plastic. My children, Willa and Georgia Cowan-Essig, make writing possible each and every day of my life because they believe that what I do is important, important enough to leave me alone for hours on end. My co-parent, Liza Cowan, was always willing to take our daughters for days on end while I traipsed off to cosmetic surgery conferences around the world or took writing retreats. My parents, Abe and Elinor Essig, are the most supportive and generous parents a person could ever have. As is the entire extended Essig clan. My family at Blue Wave Taekwondo kept me sane by letting me kick and hit them whenever I needed to. Last, but not least, I want to thank my friends Ellen Weber and Kelly Arbor. For very different reasons, they taught me everything I needed to know to write this book. They also taught me what it means to be a true friend. I hope the ties that bind us are as flexible as plastic and as strong as steel.

Notes

Introduction

1. Data on cosmetic surgery is from the Web site of the American Society of Aesthetic Plastic Surgeons, www.surgery.org, unless otherwise noted.
2. See Cele C. Otnes and Elizabeth H. Pleck, *Cinderella Dreams: The Allure of the Lavish Wedding* (Berkeley: University of California Press, 2003), especially pp. 18–19.
3. Juliet Schor, *The Overspent American: Upscaling, Downshifting, and the New Consumer* (New York: Basic Books, 1998), p. 12.
4. See Kim Khan, "How Does Your Debt Compare?" MSN Money, http://moneycentral.msn.com/content/SavingandDebt/P70581.asp; and Motley Fool, "Credit Center: Industry Secrets," www.fool.com/ccc/secrets/secrets.htm.
5. American Society of Plastic Surgeons, "Plastic Surgery Myths," www.plasticsurgery.org/Patients_and_Consumers/Plastic_Surgery_Myths.html#myth9.
6. Pierre Bourdieu, *Distinction: A Social Critique of the Judgment of Taste,* trans. Richard Nice (Cambridge, MA: Harvard University Press, 1987), p. 175.
7. Plastic surgery throughout the world is primarily performed on women. Indeed, the average percentage of female patients among plastic surgeons from all over the world is 85 percent, slightly lower than in the United States, but still overwhelmingly female. Author interviews, July 2007.
8. American Society for Aesthetic Plastic Surgery, Cosmetic Surgery National Data Bank Statistics, 2004, www.surgery.org/download/2004-stats.pdf, p. 3.
9. Rush Limbaugh, "Does Our Looks-Obsessed Culture Want to Stare at an Aging Woman?" www.rushlimbaugh.com/home/daily/site_121707/content/01125114.guest.html.guest.html, December 17, 2007.
10. Naomi Klein, *The Shock Doctrine: The Rise of Disaster Capitalism* (New York: Metropolitan Books, 2007).

Chapter 1: A Short History of Plastic

1. Partial face transplants are actually quite common. As of September 2009 there had been only nine full face transplants, but with eight of the patients surviving and in good to excellent condition, there will be more. See University of Louisville School of Medicine, Plastic Surgery Research Laboratories Web site, www.plasticsurgeryresearch.louisville.edu/index.htm.
2. Nora Jacobson*, Cleavage: Technology, Controversy, and the Irony of the Man-made Breast* (Rutgers, NJ: Rutgers University Press, 2000), p. 172.

3. Sander L. Gilman, *Making the Body Beautiful: A Cultural History of Aesthetic Surgery* (Princeton, NJ: Princeton University Press, 1999), pp. 9–10. Gilman sees aesthetic surgery as developing during the Renaissance. I argue here that it is thoroughly modern.

4. Michel Foucault, *Discipline and Punish: The Birth of the Prison* (New York: Vintage Books, 1979), p. 308.

5. Armand Marie Leroi, *Mutants: On Genetic Variety and the Human Body* (New York: Penguin Books, 2003), p. 6.

6. Rosemarie Garland Thomson, ed. *Freakery: Cultural Spectacles of the Extraordinary Body* (New York: New York University Press, 1996), p. 3.

7. Martin F. Norden and Madeleine A. Cahill, "Violence, Women, and Disability in Tod Browning's *Freaks* and *The Devil-Doll,*" *Journal of Popular Film and Television* 23 (June 1998).

8. See Gary Laderman, *Rest in Peace: A Cultural History of Death and the Funeral Home in Twentieth-century America* (New York: Oxford University Press, 2003).

9. Morton L. Berson, MD, *Atlas of Plastic Surgery* (New York: Grune and Stratton, 1948), p. i.

10. Richard Backstein and Anna Hinek, "War and Medicine: The Origins of Plastic Surgery," *Historical Review* 82, no. 3 (May 2005), p. 217.

11. Jacobson, *Cleavage,* pp. 172–73.

12. Elaine Abelson, *When Ladies Go A-Thieving: Middle-Class Shoplifters in the Victorian Department Store* (New York: Oxford University Press, 1989), p. 34.

13. Historian Elizabeth Haiken describes the birth of cosmetic surgery as "a particularly American solution to the inequalities of the modern world."

14. Anne McClintock, *Imperial Leather: Race, Gender, and Sexuality in the Colonial Context* (New York: Routledge, 1995), p. 33.

15. Vintage ad for Camay soap, available at Google Images, http://images.google.ca.

16. Rosemary Wiss, "Lipreading: Remembering Saartjie Baartman," *Australian Journal of Anthropology* 5, nos. 1–2 (1994).

17. Phillips Verner Bradford and Harvey Blume, *Ota Benga: The Pygmy in the Zoo* (New York: Bantam Doubleday, 1992).

18. Ibid., p. 118.

19. Ibid., especially pp. 126–30.

20. Sander L. Gilman, *Creating Beauty to Cure the Soul: Race and Psychology in the Shaping of Aesthetic Surgery* (Durham, NC: Duke University Press, 1998), pp. 7 and 25.

21. "The 'beautiful' becomes the 'happy.' Aesthetic surgeons operate on the body to heal the psyche. . . . The ability (and the desire) to alter the body medically for aesthetic reasons is . . . of the same vintage as modern clinical psychiatry and psychoanalysis and springs from the same desire." Ibid., p. 72; and see also p. 82.

22. Gilman, *Making the Body Beautiful,* p. 16.

23. Wendy Kline, "A New Deal for the Child," in Susan Currell and Christina Cogdell, eds., *Popular Eugenics: National Efficiency and American Mass Culture in the 1930s* (Athens: Ohio University Press, 2006), p. 23.

24. Ibid., p. 164.

25. Virginia Blum, *Flesh Wounds: The Culture of Cosmetic Surgery* (Berkeley: University of California Press, 2003), p. 3.

26. Gilman, *Making the Body Beautiful,* chapter 3, "The Racial Nose."

27. Quoted in Siobhan Somerville, *Queering the Color Line: Race and the Invention of Homosexuality* (Durham, NC: Duke University Press, 2000).

28. Anne McClintock also points out that, by the latter half of the nineteenth century, "the analogy between race and gender degeneration . . . emerged . . . the idea of racial deviance was evoked to police the 'degenerate' classes—the militant working class, the Irish, Jews, feminists, gays and lesbians, prostitutes, criminals, alcoholics and the insane—who were collectively figured as racial deviants, atavistic throwbacks to a primitive moment in human prehistory." McClintock, *Imperial Leather,* p. 43.

29. Victoria Sherrow, *For Appearance' Sake: The Encyclopedia of Good Looks, Beauty, and Grooming* (Santa Barbara, CA: Oryx Press, 2001), p. 4.

30. Marcel Mauss, "The Notion of Body Techniques," in *Sociology and Psychology: Essays,* trans. Ben Brewster (New York: Routledge & Kegan Paul, 1979), p. 100. I want to thank Graham Cassano for bringing this essay to my attention.

31. See "The Order of Simulacra" in Jean Baudrillard, *Symbolic Exchange and Death,* trans. Iain Hamilton Grant (London: Sage, 1993).

32. We need only consider how many stage actors suddenly "required" aesthetic surgery when switching to the new medium of film. Fanny Brice is a famous example; Rudolph Valentino's brother, Albert Guglielmi, despite having seven nose jobs, could never get the "right nose" for the movies. Elizabeth Haiken, *Venus Envy: A History of Cosmetic Surgery* (Baltimore: Johns Hopkins University Press, 1997), p. 97.

33. See Ibid., p. 12, and "Fanny Brice," Jewish Virtual Library, www.jewish virtuallibrary.org/jsource/biography/brice.html.

34. "I Am Woman, Hear Me Shop," *BusinessWeek,* February 14, 2005.

35. Haiken, *Venus Envy,* p. 16.

36. Ibid., p. 102.

37. Joan Jacobs Brumberg, *The Body Project: An Intimate History of American Girls* (New York: Random House, 1997), pp. 108–12.

38. M. G. Lord, *Forever Barbie: The Unauthorized Biography of a Real Doll* (New York: William Morrow and Company, 1994), p. 244.

39. Haiken, *Venus Envy,* p. 244.

40. Brumberg, *The Body Project,* p. 112; Haiken, *Venus Envy,* p. 243.

41. Nancy N. Lyons, "Interpretive Reading of Two Maidenform Bra Advertising Campaigns," *Clothing and Textiles Research Journal* 23, no. 4 (2005), p. 322.

42. Haiken, *Venus Envy,* pp. 245–57.

43. American Society of Plastic Surgeons, "The History of Plastic Surgery, ASPS and PSEF," www.plasticsurgery.org/About_ASPS/History_of_Plastic_Surgery .html#1970s.

44. www.beautyandthebreast.org.

45. www.implantsout.com.

46. Susan J. Douglas, "Where the Girls Are: Growing Up Female with the Mass Media," in Barbara A. Arrighi, ed., *Understanding Inequality: The Intersection of Race/Ethnicity, Class and Gender* (Lanham, MD: Rowman and Littlefield, 2007), p. 243.

47. Ibid., p. 222.

48. Mitra Toossi, "A Century of Change: The US Labor Force, 1950–2050," *Monthly Labor Review* 125, no. 5 (2002), p. 15.

49. Reagan always denied that her taut face was the result of surgical intervention, but *People* magazine wrote that both Nancy Reagan and Betty Ford had facelifts. Marjorie Rosen, "On the Cutting Edge," *People,* January 27, 1992.

50. Susan Faludi, *Backlash: The Undeclared War against American Women* (New York: Anchor Books, 1992), p. 228.

51. Haiken, *Venus Envy,* p. 294.

52. Ibid.

53. Cynthia L. Ogden et al., "Prevalence of Overweight and Obesity in the United States, 1999–2004," *Journal of the American Medical Association* 295, no. 13 (2006), pp. 1549–55.

54. Haiken, *Venus Envy,* p. 229.

55. Data from American Society for Aesthetic Plastic Surgery, www.surgery.org.

56. "Liposuction No Longer the Most Popular Surgical Procedure According to New Statistics," ASAPS Press Center, www.surgery.org/media/news-releases/ liposuction-no-longer-the-most-popular-surgical-procedure-according-to -new-statistics, March 16, 2009.

57. See Ylan Q. Mui, "Blue Chip, White Cotton: What Underwear Says About the Economy," *Washington Post,* August 31, 2009.

58. Simone de Beauvoir, *The Second Sex* (New York: Vintage Books, 1952), p. 592.

59. Faludi, *Backlash.*

60. I discuss Wolf's argument more fully in chapter 4. See Naomi Wolf, *The Beauty Myth: How Images of Beauty Are Used against Women* (New York: William Morrow, 1991).

61. Kathy Davis, *Reshaping the Female Body: The Dilemma of Cosmetic Surgery* (New York: Routledge, 1995).

62. Deborah Coslav Covino, *Amending the Abject Body: Aesthetic Makeovers in Medicine and Culture* (Albany, NY: State University of New York Press, 2004), p. 13.

63. Debra L. Gimlin, *Body Work: Beauty and Self-Image in American Culture* (Berkeley: University of California Press, 2002), p. 2.

64. Anthony Elliot, *Making the Cut: How Cosmetic Surgery Is Transforming Our Lives* (London: Reaktion Books 2008), pp. 19 and 46.

65. "For Americans and for their cosmetic surgeons, the individual, external self offers a last and apparently everlasting frontier." Haiken, *Venus Envy*, pp. 300–301.

Chapter 2: The State of Plastic

1. Hoover Institution, Stanford University, "Facts on Policy: Consumer Spending," www.hoover.org/research/factsonpolicy/facts/4931661.html.

2. Jose Garcia, James Lardner, and Cindy Zeldin, *Up to Our Eyeballs: How Shady Lenders and Failed Economic Policies Are Drowning Americans in Debt* (New York: New Press, 2008), p. 33.

3. Ruth Simon and James R. Hagerty, "Delayed Foreclosures Stalk Market," *Wall Street Journal,* September 23, 2009.

4. Ibid., pp. 57–61.

5. For an excellent discussion of Friedman and his legacy, see Naomi Klein, *The Shock Doctrine: The Rise of Disaster Capitalism* (New York: Henry Holt, 2007).

6. David Harvey, *A Brief History of Neoliberalism* (New York: Oxford University Press, 2005), p. 7.

7. Ronald Reagan speech to schoolchildren, November 1988, quoted in Matt Gertz, "Conservative Media Take Note: Reagan Preached Tax Cut Gospel to America's Students," Media Matters for America, www.mediamatters.org.

8. See Robert Lekachman, *Greed Is Not Enough: Reaganomics* (New York: Pantheon, 1982).

9. American Political Science Association, Task Force on Inequality and American Democracy, www.apsanet.org/content_2471.cfm.

10. Robert D. Manning, *Credit Card Nation: The Consequences of America's Addiction to Credit* (New York: Basic Books, 2000), p. 60.

11. www.neoperspectives.com/RonaldReagan.htm.

12. Jeremy Howell and Alan Ingham, "From Social Problem to Personal Issue: The Language of Lifestyle," *Cultural Studies* 15, no. 2 (2001), pp. 326–51.

13. Frank says that neoliberal beliefs from below, what he calls the Great Backlash, "is what has made possible the international free-market consensus of recent years, with all the privatization, deregulation, and deunionization that are its components. Backlash ensures that Republicans will continue to be returned to office even when their free-market miracles fail and their libertarian schemes don't deliver and their 'New Economy' collapses." Thomas

Frank, *What's the Matter with Kansas? How Conservatives Won the Heart of America* (New York: Metropolitan Books, 2004), p. 5.

14. Robert H. Frank, *Falling Behind: How Rising Inequality Harms the Middle Class* (Berkeley: University of California Press, 2007), p. 48.

15. Elizabeth Haiken, *Venus Envy: A History of Cosmetic Surgery* (Baltimore: Johns Hopkins University Press, 1997), p. 294.

16. Deborah A. Sullivan, *Cosmetic Surgery: The Cutting Edge of Commercial Medicine in America* (New Brunswick, NJ: Rutgers University Press, 2001).

17. www.plasticsurgery.org/x6156.xml?prid=22&caseid=8564.

18. www.angelslab.com/cosmetic-plastic-surgery-computer-imaging.asp.

19. North Dallas Plastic Surgery Web site, http://drpollock.com/before-and -after-pictures.htm.

20. Robert Roy Britt, "Cosmetic Surgery Expected to Soar," *Live Science,* June 24, 2008.

21. "Plastic Surgery Financing," www.makemeheal.com/mmh/surgery_financing/ index.vm.

22. Consumer Guide to Plastic Surgery, www.yourplasticsurgeryguide.com/trends/ demographic-changes.htm.

23. Manning, *Credit Card Nation,* p. 11.

24. Garcia, Lardner, and Zeldin, *Up to Our Eyeballs,* p. 31.

25. Marshall Eckblad, "In Banks' Profit Push, 'Era of Low Fees Is Over,'" *Wall Street Journal,* July 31, 2009.

26. Garcia, Lardner, and Zeldin, *Up to Our Eyeballs*, p. 144.

27. Brian Grow and Robert Berner, "Fresh Pain for the Uninsured," *BusinessWeek,* November 21, 2007.

28. Ibid. For more on how the economic downturn shaped this thriving credit industry, see chapter 6.

29. www.carecredit.com.

30. Garcia, Lardner, and Zeldin, *Up to Our Eyeballs,* pp. 135–37.

31. Zachary A. Goldfarb and Alejandro Lazo, "Capital One's Profit Plunges 40 Percent," *Washington Post,* July 18, 2008.

32. Based on my interviews with plastic surgeons at the International Confederation for Plastic, Reconstructive, and Aesthetic Surgery (IPRAS) conference in Berlin, July 2007.

Chapter 3: Plastic People and Their Doctors

1. Virginia L. Blum, *Flesh Wounds: The Culture of Cosmetic Surgery* (Berkeley: University of California Press, 2003), p. 23.

2. L. Neumayer et al., "Perceptions of Women Medical Students and Their Influence on Career Choice," *American Journal of Surgery* 183, no. 2 (2002), p. 146.

3. According to an organizer of ASAPS conferences, about 90 percent of the plastic surgeons who attend are men.

4. These numbers actually refer to academic surgeons. Numbers for residents are slightly more representative of the U.S. population; numbers for tenured surgical professors much less representative. Paris D. Butler, Michael T. Longaker, and L. D. Britt, "Major Deficit in the Number of Underrepresented Minority Academic Surgeons Persists," *Annals of Surgery* 248, no. 5 (2008), p. 704.

5. Upward mobility between generations is lower in the United States than in Canada, Sweden, Germany, Spain, Denmark, Austria, Norway, Finland, and France. At the same time, the nation's colleges and universities, a major engine for social and economic mobility, became less affordable for working families. Between 2004 and 2006, for example, college affordability declined in seventeen states, and need-based student aid badly failed to keep pace. There are many reports on the increasing economic insecurity among the vast majority of Americans. For instance, see the 2006 report of the Opportunity Agenda, a nonprofit think tank: *The State of Opportunity,* www.opportunityagenda .org. See also the Federal Reserve Board's data at www.federalreserve.gov/ pubs/ feds/2006/200613/200613pap.pdf.

6. C. Wright Mills, *The Sociological Imagination* (New York: Oxford University Press, 1959; rev. ed. 2000).

7. Grace Wong, "Ka-ching! Wedding Price Tag Nears $30K," CNNMoney. com, money.cnn.com/2005/05/20/pf/weddings, May 20, 2005. For more on the role of the ideology of romance in American culture, see Chrys Ingraham, *White Weddings: Romancing Heterosexuality in Popular Culture* (New York: Routledge, 1999), and Cele C. Otnes and Elisabeth H. Pleck, *Cinderella Dreams: The Allure of the Lavish Wedding* (Berkeley and Los Angeles: University of California Press, 2003).

8. It is interesting to note that the last U.S. president to not have a spouse was James Buchanan (1857–61).

9. U.S. Census Bureau, "Unmarried and Single Americans Week," Facts for Figures Special Edition press release, July 19, 2004, www.census.gov/Press -Release/www/releases/archives/facts_for_features_special_editions/002265 .html; and Centers for Disease Control and Prevention, *National Vital Statistics Reports* 48, no. 1 (2000), www.cdc.gov/nchs/data/nvsr/nvsr48/nvs48_01.pdf. In fact, divorce rates are not quite 50 percent; more like 43 percent of marriages will end in divorce in the first fifteen years of marriage. Still, the chances of never marrying or of being divorced are quite high for most Americans.

10. Deborah Davis and Michael L. Vernon, "Sculpting the Body Beautiful: Attachment Style, Neuroticism, and the Use of Cosmetic Surgeries," *Sex Roles* 47, nos. 3–4 (2002), p. 136.

11. "Dramatic Changes in U.S. Aging Highlighted in New Census, NIH Report," *NIH News,* March 9, 2006, www.nih.gov/news/pr/mar2006/nia-09.htm.

12. Malcolm Gladwell, *The Tipping Point: How Little Things Can Make a Big Difference* (Boston: Little, Brown, 2000).

13. In the fall of 2008, a plastic surgeon acquaintance agreed to send out ten letters asking his colleagues to let me interview them. Not a single one even responded to say no. Not even after a follow-up reminder was sent. Thus I had to rely on the interviews I conducted at the professional conferences. The limitation to these interviews is that not every doctor conducting plastic surgery is a member of a professional organization like ASAPS, especially since no particular qualifications beyond a medical degree are required to perform cosmetic surgery.

14. American Medical Association, www.ama-assn.org/ama/pub.

15. Natasha Singer, "For Top Medical Students, An Attractive Field," *New York Times,* March 19, 2008.

16. Deborah A. Sullivan, *Cosmetic Surgery: The Cutting Edge of Commercial Medicine in America* (New Brunswick, NJ: Rutgers University Press, 2001), p. 81.

17. Elizabeth Haiken, "The Making of the Modern Face," *Social Research* 67, no. 1 (2000), p. 93.

Chapter 4: Learning to Be Plastic: Magazines, TV, and Other Cultural Scripts

1. Maya Angelou, "On Reaching Forty," *Poems* (New York: Bantam Books, 1986), p. 58.

2. Rich Cohen, "Madonnarama!" *Vanity Fair,* May 2008.

3. Joan Rivers, with Valerie Frankel, *Men Are Stupid . . . And They Like Big Boobs: A Woman's Guide to Beauty Through Plastic Surgery* (New York: Pocket Books, 2009).

4. Joan Jacobs Brumberg, *The Body Project: An Intimate History of American Girls* (New York: Random House, 1997), pp. xvii–xx.

5. Nannette Magruder Pratt, *The Body Beautiful: Common-Sense Ideas on Health and Beauty without Medicine* (New York: Baker and Taylor, 1902).

6. Max Weber, *The Protestant Ethic and the Spirit of Capitalism and Other Writings* (New York: Penguin Books, 2002).

7. Micki McGee, *Self Help, Inc.: Makeover Culture in American Life* (New York: Oxford University Press, 2005).

8. Susan Bordo, *Unbearable Weight: Feminism, Western Culture, and the Body* (Berkeley: University of California Press, 1993), pp. 245–46.

9. See Joke Hermes, *Reading Women's Magazines: An Analysis of Everyday Media Use* (Cambridge, MA: Polity, 1996).

10. Andrea N. Polonijo et al. "Representations of Cosmetic Surgery and Emotional Health in Women's Magazines in Canada," *Women's Health Issues* 18, no. 6 (2008), p. 463.

11. Information from *O, The Oprah Magazine* media kit.

12. Author's interview with Joan Kron, June 2009.

13. *Allure* mission statement, www.condenastmediakit.com/all/index.cfm.

14. Michael Shields, "Mag Spotlight: New Beauty," *Media Daily News,* December 17, 2004, www.mediapost.com/publications.

15. Kathryn Lofton, "Practicing Oprah; or, the Prescriptive Compulsion of a Spiritual Capitalism," *Journal of Popular Culture* 39, no. 4 (2006), pp. 599–621.

16. I looked at the January–May 2004, January–October 2007, and February–June 2009 issues of *O, The Oprah Magazine. O* magazine was usually 250-plus pages, with slightly more than one-third devoted to advertisements. Ads for anti-aging skin creams averaged six per issue. Ads for cosmetic procedures (usually Botox or Juvéderm) appeared in most issues after February 2004. There was usually one article per issue after February 2004 about cosmetic procedures, generally under the heading "Beauty."

17. I looked at the January–June 2009 issues of *Allure.* The images of women in *Allure* are also nearly all white (the pop singer Rihanna was the only non-white woman to grace its cover in the year I looked at *Allure,* and nearly all the women in the ads and articles are white).

18. *Allure,* June 2009.

19. Joan Kron, "Clock Stoppers, Skin Tricks," *Allure,* January 8, 2008.

20. I looked at summer/fall 2007 through summer/fall 2008 issues of *New Beauty.*

21. Joan Kron, *Lift: Wanting, Fearing, and Having a Facelift* (New York: Penguin Books, 1998).

22. Author's interview, May 21, 2009.

23. One of the earlier studies to demonstrate a link between ideal types and self-satisfaction was Marsha L. Richins, "Social Comparison and the Idealized Images of Advertising," *Journal of Consumer Research* 18, no. 1 (1991), pp. 71–83.

24. www.drrobertrey.com/dr-90210.htm.

25. Sarah Banet-Weiser and Laura Portwood-Stacer, "'I just want to be me again!' Beauty Pageants, Reality Television and Post-Feminism," *Feminist Theory* 7, no. 2 (2006), p. 263.

26. Maria Elena Fernandez, "For 'Nip/Tuck' Beauty Fades," *Los Angeles Times,* June 20, 2009.

27. Sue Tait, a lecturer at the University of Canterbury, considers how effective *Nip/Tuck* is at criticizing cosmetic surgery, and finds that although the show does present feminist frames of surgery, it does so through individual characters and therefore never really provides the possibility of a coherent collective

movement against an unavoidably surgical culture. Sue Tait, "Television and the Domestication of Cosmetic Surgery," *Feminist Media Studies* 7, no. 2 (2007), pp. 119–35.

28. Quoted on DVD bonus feature, *Nip/Tuck* season 2, released August 30, 2005.

29. Quoted in Natasha Singer, "Skin Deep; A Doctor? He Is One on TV," *New York Times,* March 16, 2006.

30. Richard J. Crockett et al., "The Influence of Plastic Surgery 'Reality TV' on Cosmetic Surgery Patient Expectations and Decision Making," *Plastic and Reconstructive Surgery* 120, no. 1 (July 2007).

31. American Society for Aesthetic and Plastic Surgery, "America's Approval of Cosmetic Surgery at an All-Time High," press release, March 9, 2007.

32. For instance, see Marsha L. Richins, "Social Comparison and the Idealized Images of Advertising," *Journal of Consumer Research* 18, no. 1 (1991), pp. 71–83.

33. Rivers, *Men Are Stupid,* p. 23.

Chapter 5: The Mirror and the Porn Star: Ideal Forms, Cosmetic Surgery, and Everyday Aesthetics

1. www.wikihow.com/Look-Like-a-Pornstar.

2. Without rehashing the anti-porn arguments too much, it seems worth pointing out that the claim was that porn did not just represent violence against women, but constituted action. In other words, it was like yelling "Fire!" in a crowded theater, because it caused people to act in certain ways. For instance, see Catharine A. MacKinnon, "Pornography, Civil Rights, and Speech," *Harvard Civil Rights–Civil Liberties Law Review* 1 (1985), and "Turning Rape into Pornography: Postmodern Genocide," *Ms., July/August 1993.

3. Pat Califia, "The Obscene, Disgusting, and Vile Meese Commission Report," in *Public Sex: The Culture of Radical Sex* (Pittsburgh: Cleis Press, 1994).

4. http://thinkexist.com/quotes/ron_jeremy.

5. Jeff Langenderfer and Steven W. Kopp, "The Digital Technology Revolution and Its Effect on Copyrighted Works," *Journal of Macromarketing* 24, no. 1 (2004), p. 17.

6. Of course, the private/female versus the public/male divisions have always been highly contested and therefore constantly negotiated and renegotiated. For more on public/private spaces and pornography, see Danielle de Voss, "Women's Porn Sites: Spaces of Fissure and Eruption or 'I'm a Little Bit of Everything,'" *Sexuality and Culture* 6, no. 3 (June 2002).

7. Violet Blue, "Are More Women OK with Watching Porn?" *O, The Oprah Magazine,* July 1, 2007.

8. Rebecca Leung, "Porn in the USA," *Sixty Minutes,* September 5, 2004, www

.cbsnews.com/stories/2003/11/21/60minutes/main585049.shtml. This fig-ure has been disputed by some. See Dan Ackman, "How Big Is Porn?" *Forbes,* May 25, 2001, www.forbes.com/2001/05/25/0524porn.html. That the in-dustry was the first to figure out how to profit from the VCR and now the Internet is undisputed.

9. Joe Mandese, "Media Metrics: Porn: Stickier Than You Think," *MediaPost,* July 1, 2005, http://publications.mediapost.com/index.cfm?fuseaction=Articles .showArticle&art_aid=31463.

10. There are, at this point, many books on the pornification of modern life, in-cluding Susanna Passonen, Kaarina Nikunen, and Laura Saarenmaa, *Pornifica-tion: Sex and Sexuality in Media Culture* (New York: Berg, 2007), and Carmine Sarracino and Kevin M. Scott, *The Porning of America: The Rise of American Porn Culture, What It Means, and Where We Go from Here* (Boston: Beacon Press, 2008).

11. Linda Williams, *Porn Studies* (Durham, NC: Duke University Press, 2004), p. 3.

12. David Wallechinsky and Irving Wallace, *The People's Almanac* (New York: Doubleday, 1975).

13. CNN, "Playboy Founder Hefner, 82, Talks of Empire, Girlfriends," January 9, 2009, CNN.com.

14. P. T. Katzmarzyk and C. Davis, "Thinness and Body Shape of *Playboy* Center-folds from 1978 to 1998," *International Journal of Obesity* 25, no. 4 (2001).

15. It's worth noting that many of the earlier Playmates may have had nose jobs. This fact was pointed out to me by a plastic surgeon friend, Chris McEwan, who gallantly offered to look over my collection of Playmates for his expert opinion on what cosmetic procedures were evident. Dr. McEwan did note, however, that it is only after 1985 that all of the Playmates I showed him had some form of cosmetic intervention.

16. www.sonypictures.com/homevideo/thehousebunny/index.html.

17. www.hottopic.com.

18. www.forthegirls.com.

19. www.sssh.com.

20. "Porn for Ladies: What Do They Like?" *Ecommerce Journal,* July 21, 2009.

21. Terrie Schauer, "Women's Porno: The Heterosexual Female Gaze in Porn Sites 'For Women,'" *Sexuality and Culture* 9, no. 2 (2005), pp. 57–59.

22. American Society of Plastic Surgeons, "2007 Quick Facts: Cosmetic and Re-constructive Plastic Surgery Trends," www.plasticsurgery.org.

23. Laser Vaginal Rejuvenation Institute of Los Angeles, www.drmatlock.com.

24. Leonore Tiefer, "Female Genital Cosmetic Surgery: Freakish or Inevitable? Analysis from Medical Marketing, Bioethics, and Feminist Theory," *Feminism and Psychology* 18 (2008), p. 466.

25. Author's interview, February 2007.

26. Phit MedSpa, www.theperfectphit.com/.

27. Naomi Wolf, "The Porn Myth," *New York Magazine*, November 26, 2007, http://nymag.com/nymetro/news/trends/n_9437/.

28. Nancy Etcoff, *Survival of the Prettiest: The Science of Beauty* (New York: Anchor, 2000), p. 74.

29. See, for example, Jacquelyn Dowd Hall, *Revolt against Chivalry* (New York: Columbia University Press, 1993); Grace Elizabeth Hale, *Making Whiteness: The Culture of Segregation in the South, 1890–1940* (New York: Vintage, 1999); Anne McClintock, *Imperial Leather: Race, Gender, and Sexuality in the Colonial Contest* (New York: Routledge, 1995); Siobhan Somerville, *Queering the Color Line: Race and the Invention of Homosexuality in American Culture* (Durham, NC: Duke University Press, 2000); and Judith Walkowitz, *City of Dreadful Delight: Narratives of Sexual Danger in Late-Victorian London* (Chicago: University of Chicago Press, 1992).

30. Quoted in Somerville, *Queering the Color Line*, pp. 27–28.

31. James Kincaid, *Erotic Innocence: The Culture of Child Molesting* (Durham, NC: Duke University Press, 1998).

32. Michael Mehta and Dwaine Plaza, "Pornography in Cyberspace," in *Culture of the Internet*, ed. Sarah Kiesler (Mahwah, NJ: Laurence Erlbaum, 1997).

33. Andrew Dillon, "Reading from Paper versus Screens: A Critical View of the Empirical Literature," *Ergonomics* 35, no. 10 (1992).

34. www.myfreeimplants.com.

Chapter 6: Broken Plastic

1. "Fantastic Plastic Changes Color When It's Stretched to the Breaking Point," Discovermagazine.com, 80beats Blog, May 7, 2009, http://blogs.discover-magazine.com/80beats/2009/05/07/fantastic-plastic-changes-color-when-its-stretched-to-the-breaking-point/.

2. U.S. Department of Labor, Bureau of Labor Statistics, www.bls.gov.

3. Jeffrey Frankel, a Harvard economist and member of the Business Cycle Dating Committee of the National Bureau of Economic Research, called it a depression. Scott Thill, "The Robber Barons Are Back—Hide Your Money!" AlterNet, October 19, 2009.

4. S. Mitra Kalita, "The 'Democratization of Credit' Is Over—Now It's Payback Time," *Wall Street Journal*, October 10, 2009.

5. Pippa Wysong, "The Price of Looking Good in the Credit Crunch: An Expert Interview with Sherell J. Aston, MD, FACS," *Medscape Today*, June 17, 2009.

6. Natasha Singer, "Vanity's Downturn: Botox Use, and Allergan Sales, Dip," *New York Times*, February 4, 2009.

7. Laurie Essig, "Ordinary Ugliness: The Hidden Cost of the Credit Crunch," *Chronicle of Higher Education,* January 30, 2009.

8. American Society for Aesthetic Plastic Surgery, 2008 Statistics on Cosmetic Surgery.

9. Cosmetic Surgery Plastic Research, "Statistics and Trends," www.cosmetic plasticsurgerystatistics.com/statistics.html#2007-NEWS.

10. Actually, there are no good data on surgery rates internationally. The International Confederation for Plastic, Reconstructive, and Aesthetic Surgery (IP-RAS) is the largest international body of cosmetic and reconstructive surgeons, but it is a voluntary organization and thus its data do not represent actual rates of cosmetic surgery.

11. British Association of Aesthetic Plastic Surgeons, "Cosmetic Rates of Inflation: Male, Female Breast Ops on the Rise," www.baaps.org.uk/about-us/press-releases/453-cosmetic-rates-of-inflation-male-female-breast-ops-on-the-rise.

12. *RealtyTrac* staff, "Sun Belt Cities Top List of Nation's Metro Foreclosure Rates in First Quarter," *RealtyTrac,* April 22, 2009.

13. Brian Wargo, "Las Vegas Economy in Free Fall," *Las Vegas Sun,* March 13, 2009.

14. Tom Hertz, *Understanding Mobility in America* (Washington, DC: Center for American Progress, 2006).

15. Barbara Ehrenreich, *Bait and Switch: The (Futile) Pursuit of the American Dream* (New York: Metropolitan Books, 2005).

16. Unlike the two previous recessions, the Great Recession is actually hurting working-class (especially Black) people more than white-collar workers (although this may change in the future since much of the pain stems from job losses in the construction industry, but the collapsed home values will eventually hurt the owning classes more than renters). It's possible that the white-collar patients really do see their unemployment as temporary and as offering them a chance to get cosmetic work done before they get their next job. Howard J. Wall, *The Effects of Recessions Across Demographic Groups* (Federal Reserve Bank of St. Louis, September 2009).

17. For instance, a poll released in October 2009 conducted for the nonprofit Americans for Financial Reform showed most Americans wanted more regulation of credit and complex financial products like derivatives. Those polled saw the lack of regulation as the cause of the financial crisis. See Americans for Financial Reform, "Recent Polling Data on Financial Reform Regulation," http://ourfinancialsecurity.org/2009/10/recent-polling-data-on-financial-reform-legislation/.

18. George Gohl, "Showdown in Chicago: Creating a 'Which Side Are You On?' Moment," Huffington Post, October 22, 2009.

19. Art Levine, "The Battle against Letting Wall Street Continue to Make a Killing on Derivatives," AlterNet, October 21, 2009.

20. Victoria McGrane, "The Early Returns on the CFPA Vote," Politico, October 23, 2009.

21. U.S. Chamber of Commerce, "Vote for Business," http://capwiz.com/chamber/issues/alert/?alertid=13947486.

22. Paul Wiseman, "Industry Lines Up to Fight Consumer Protection Agency," *USA Today,* September 14, 2009.

23. "Schwarzenegger Tightens Cosmetic Surgery Laws," *Economic Times,* October 21, 2009.

24. This includes laws like the Riegle-Neal Interstate Banking and Branching Efficiency Act and the Gramm-Leach-Bliley Act. Margot Saunders and Alys Cohen, *Federal Regulation of Consumer Credit: The Cause or Cure for Predatory Lending?* (Cambridge, MA: Harvard University Joint Center for Housing Studies, March 2004).

25. Alyx Kuczynski gives a hilarious and harrowing account of a medical tourism trip to South Africa in *Beauty Junkies: Inside Our $15 Billion Obsession with Cosmetic Surgery* (New York: Doubleday, 2006), pp. 22–35.

26. www.navigateglobalhealth.com.

27. Natasha Singer, "Beauty on the Black Market," *New York Times,* February 16, 2006.

28. "Death Exposes Illegal Cosmetic Surgery Network," MSNBC.com, September 7, 2006.

29. "Priscilla Presley's Mug Is Too Full," *New York Daily News,* March 25, 2008.

30. "FDA Law Enforcers Crack Down on Illegal Botox Scammers," Consumer Health Information, www.fda.gov/consumer.

Chapter 7: Resistance

1. David Moos, "Memories of Being: Orlan's Theater of the Self," *Art + Text* 54 (1996), pp. 67–72; Theresa M. Senft, "Feminism, Technology, Performance," Women and New Media Panel, Women and the Arts Conference, Rutgers University, May 18, 1998, www.terrisenft.net/writing/rutgers.html.

2. Catherine Dunn, *Geek Love* (New York: Knopf, 1989).

3. Tim Bayne and Neil Levy, "Amputees By Choice," *Journal of Applied Philosophy* 22, no. 1 (2005).

4. Michael First, "Desire for Amputation of a Limb: Paraphilia, Psychosis, or a New Type of Identity Disorder," *Psychological Medicine* 35, no. 6 (2005), pp. 919–28.

5. www.transabled.org.

6. *Whole,* a documentary by Melody Gilbert and FRZN Productions (2003), follows several amputee wannabes (and some who have become successful

amputees) through their daily lives. The people in the film explain themselves to an audience of skeptics, no doubt, but they do so in the language of rationality, choice, and innate and unchanging identities.

7. www.thelizardman.com.

8. "Tiger Man Wants Fur Graft," *Guardian,* August 2, 2001, www.guardian .co.uk/silly/story/0,10821,531386,00.html.

9. www.stalkingcat.net.

10. Vanessa Renee Casavant, "Catman's Transformation Raises Concerns over Extreme Surgery," *Seattle Times,* August 16, 2005.

11. www.stalkingcat.net. Another famous transspeciesist is Tom Leppard, aka the Leopard Man. Leppard was long the reigning champion of the *Guinness Book of World Records* as "the most tattooed man in the world." Sadly for Mr. Leppard, the 99.2 percent of his body covered with leopard-like spots no longer qualifies him as the most tattooed man in the world, but his many years of living a "primitive" life as half cat, half man on the shores of Loch na Bieste brought him attention from audiences around the world. Neil Stephen, "The Cat Who Came In from the Cold," *Guardian,* October 28, 2008.

12. Jeff Woloson, "Jocelyne Wildenstein," www.divasthesite.com/Society_Divas/ jocelyne_wildenstein_a.htm.

13. "Bloated Bride of Wildenstein Looks Scarier Than Ever," *Daily Mail,* September 16, 2009.

14. *Diagnostic and Statistical Manual of Mental Disorders,* 4th ed., *(DSM-IV)* (Arlington, VA: American Psychiatric Association, 2000).

15. Interview with the author, December 2005; the source wished to remain anonymous.

16. The population of the city I describe (Burlington, Vermont) is easily determined. But how to estimate the number of gender queer, female-bodied persons is much more difficult. I have done fieldwork among trans communities here since March 2005, and based on public events such as the Translating Identity Conference and Trans Day of Remembrance, there are several hundred trans people. Some of these people identify as transsexual, but one of my informants guesses that only about 20 percent of the trans community uses the term "transsexual." The rest prefer "trans" or "gender queer."

17. Indeed, something like 85 percent of cosmetic procedures in the United States are now paid for on credit, with interest rates often as high as 25 percent. The fact that credit is available to nearly everyone who walks into a surgeons' office has changed cosmetic surgery from a luxury item for the well-off to a "must-have" for a lot of Americans. A 2005 poll conducted by the American Society of Plastic Surgeons found that 30 percent of plastic surgery

patients earned less than $30,000 a year, while another 41 percent earned between $31,000 and $60,000. "Demographic Changes Among Plastic Surgery Patients," *Health on the Net,* accessed at http://www.yourplasticsurgery guide.com/trends/demographic-changes.htm.

18. Kate Bornstein's most widely cited book is *Gender Outlaw: On Men, Women, and the Rest of Us* (New York: Routledge, 1994). According to "hir" Web site, Bornstein is an author and performance artist who grew up a boy, became a man, then became a woman, then decided that being a woman didn't feel any more comfortable than being a man, and thus refused to be one or the other. See www.katebornstein.com.

19. See Judith Butler, *Gender Trouble: Feminism and the Subversion of Identity* (New York: Routledge, 1990).

20. This may or may not be true, but the stories most certainly appeared regularly. For instance, see Tom Liddy, "Jacko's Fake Nose 'Missing,'" *New York Post,* July 24, 2009.

21. "The 15 Worst Celebrity Plastic Surgery Disasters You Will Ever See," www.topsocialite.com, September 27, 2007.

22. "Tara Reid Strips for *Playboy,* Calls Lipo Scars Her 'Battle Wounds," Huffington Post, October 9, 2009.

23. "Star Jones Cheats Death As She Undergoes Plastic Surgery," *National Enquirer,* March 21, 2006.

24. "The World's Worst Plastic Surgery," *Maxim,* September 21, 2009, www.maxim.com/humor/lists/43917/worlds-worst-plastic-surgery.html?p=2.

25. "Janice Dickinson—Good and Bad Plastic Surgery," www.topsocialite.com, January 27, 2009.

26. Dr. Franz-Hubert Robling, "The Force of Plasticity: Some Reflections on the Concept of Rhetorical Subjectivity in the Works of Friedrich Nietzsche," www.uni-tuebingen.de/uni/nas/dozenten/rob-nietzsch.htm. Thank you to Gunther Roth for bringing this essay to my attention.

27. Michel de Certeau, *The Practice of Everyday Life* (Berkeley: University of California Press, 1984), p. xix.

Chapter 8: . . . Is Futile?

1. Nancy Etcoff, *Survival of the Prettiest: The Science of Beauty* (New York: Anchor Books, 1999).

2. Gordon L. Patzer, *The Power and Paradox of Physical Attractiveness* (Boca Raton, FL: Brown Walker Press), p. 66.

3. Gordon L. Patzer, *Looks: Why They Matter More Than You Ever Imagined* (New York: Amacom, 2008), p. 13.

4. Patzer and Etcoff's claims that men are inevitably attracted to young women not only leaves out homoerotic men, but also the apparently growing number of men who prefer older women, popularly referred to as "cougars." For instance, a recent news article talked about the fact that far more young men want to date older women than older women want to date young men. See Marcelle S. Fischler, "In Cougar Territory, Cubs Take the Lead," *New York Times,* November 14, 2009.

5. Rinah Yamamoto et al., "Gender Differences in the Motivational Processing of Babies Are Determined by Their Facial Attractiveness," *PloS One* 4, no. 6 (June 24, 2009).

6. Jeffrey Kluger, "Is an Ugly Baby Harder to Love?" *Time,* June 24, 2009.

7. *Amateur Scientist,* June 26, 2009.

8. *The Simpsons,* "Husbands and Knives," season 19, episode 7.

9. www.missplastichungary.com.

10. www.beautyforlife.com.

11. In the November 2009 edition of the journal *Clinical Risk,* French plastic surgeons discuss why new regulations were put into place, and British plastic surgeons discuss the need for increased state regulation of aesthetic surgery practices and advertising. *Clinical Risk* 15, no. 6.

12. "Women 'Suffer Poor Self-Esteem Due to Airbrushing in Advertising,'" *Telegraph,* November 27, 2009.

13. The American College of Obstetricians and Gynecologists took a public stance against "designer vagina" surgeries in 2007. Judith Graham, "Women Urged to Shun Trendy Plastic Surgery. Doctors Assail Genital Procedures," *Chicago Tribune,* August 31, 2007.

14. New View Campaign, "Vulvagraphics: An Intervention in Honor of Female Genital Diversity," www.newviewcampaign.org/vulvagraphics.asp.

15. Author's interview, November 2009.

16. Barbara Ehrenreich, *Bright-Sided: How the Relentless Promotion of Positive Thinking Has Undermined America* (New York: Metropolitan Books, 2009), p. 196.

17. Ronald Bailey, "The Methuselah Manifesto," *Reason,* November 17, 2009.

18. Bill Jay, "Why the Future Doesn't Need Us," *Wired,* August 2004, www.wired.com/wired/archive/8.04/joy_pr.html.

19. Erving Goffman, *The Presentation of Self in Everyday Life* (New York: Anchor Books, 1959).

Index

activist feminism, 19
advertising: for aesthetic procedures, 52, 55, 60, 94–95, 98, 181; before and after photos, 36–37, 71; and beauty, 8–10, 110, 174, 175; influence on women, 9, 17, 19, 21–22, 93–98; influence on working class, 9–10, 38–39, 41; medical, 19, 25, 30, 33, 35–38; and perfection, xiii; by physicians, 19, 25, 30, 33, 35–38; plastic magazine, 94; for plastic surgery aimed at children, 60, 74, 120, 178–79; and prestigious imitation, 14–15, 16–17, 110; wish fulfillment, 9, 17, 19, 21–22, 52, 55, 74, 93–98
aestheticians, 21, 136
African Americans: assimilating through cosmetic surgery, xx, 10, 12–13, 15, 174; demographics of O magazine, 93; view of African American women, 101, 131. See also race
aging: baby boomers, 57–59; cultural scripts about, 59, 83–86, 102, 130; historical attitudes toward, 87–89; and ordinary ugliness, 9–10, 83–84, 99, 106, 109; and plastic magazines, 94–95, 97–98; as a problem to be solved, xix–xx, 43–44, 57–59, 83, 95–98, 105; recreated as a medical condition, 52; and revulsion,

xix–xx, 71–72, 83–84, 94–96; and romance, 56–57; and sexual desire, 129, 130–32, 133; in the twenty-first century, 58; view of, in pornography, 121–22, 127
Allure magazine, 92, 93, 94–95, 97
AMA. See American Medical Association (AMA)
Amateur Scientist, 177
Amending the Abject Body (Covino), 22
American identity, xxi–xxii, 27, 34–35, 47
American Medical Association (AMA), 19, 35, 65, 128
American optimism bias, xvii–xviii, 16, 24, 30, 44, 142
American Political Science Association's Task Force on Inequality and American Democracy, 32
American Recovery and Reinvestment Act of 2009, xxi
American Society for Aesthetic Plastic Surgery (ASAPS), xiii, 20, 49–50, 110, 136
American Society of Plastic Surgeons (ASPS), xvi, 36, 38, 39, 136
amputee wannabes, 156–59
Angels Lab (Web site), 36
animal/human hybrids, 159–62
anti-elitist rhetoric, 33
anti-pornography feminism, 113
appearance and power, xx–xxi, 4, 6, 10, 17, 22
Arturism, 156–57